Necessary Conversations

The Robert Wood Johnson Foundation Culture of Health Series
Series Editor, Alonzo L. Plough

Necessary Conversations

Understanding Racism as a Barrier to Achieving Health Equity

EDITED BY ALONZO L. PLOUGH

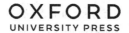

OXFORD
UNIVERSITY PRESS

OXFORD
UNIVERSITY PRESS

Oxford University Press is a department of the University of Oxford. It furthers
the University's objective of excellence in research, scholarship, and education
by publishing worldwide. Oxford is a registered trade mark of Oxford University
Press in the UK and certain other countries.

Published in the United States of America by Oxford University Press
198 Madison Avenue, New York, NY 10016, United States of America.

© Robert Wood Johnson Foundation 2022

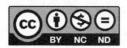
CIP data is on file at the Library of Congress
ISBN 978–0–19–764147–7

DOI: 10.1093/oso/9780197641477.001.0001

This material is not intended to be, and should not be considered, a substitute for medical or other
professional advice. Treatment for the conditions described in this material is highly dependent on the
individual circumstances. And, while this material is designed to offer accurate information with respect
to the subject matter covered and to be current as of the time it was written, research and knowledge about
medical and health issues is constantly evolving and dose schedules for medications are being revised
continually, with new side effects recognized and accounted for regularly. Readers must therefore always
check the product information and clinical procedures with the most up-to-date published product
information and data sheets provided by the manufacturers and the most recent codes of conduct and safety
regulation. The publisher and the authors make no representations or warranties to readers, express or
implied, as to the accuracy or completeness of this material. Without limiting the foregoing, the publisher
and the authors make no representations or warranties as to the accuracy or efficacy of the drug dosages
mentioned in the material. The authors and the publisher do not accept, and expressly disclaim, any
responsibility for any liability, loss, or risk that may be claimed or incurred as a consequence of the use and/
or application of any of the contents of this material.

1 3 5 7 9 8 6 4 2

Printed by Marquis, Canada

CONTENTS

ACKNOWLEDGMENTS

The *Sharing Knowledge* conference involved the hard work of many talented individuals, both internal and external to the Robert Wood Johnson Foundation. Tracy Costigan and Martina Todaro led the successful development of the conference.

Turning the fifth annual conference into this volume also required the vision and support of many. An Editorial Review Group oversees the development of this series and provided careful commentary and suggestions. My colleagues in this group are Sandro Galea, Boston University; Sherry Glied, New York University; Anita Chandra, RAND Corporation; and Sarah Humphreville, Oxford University Press.

Special thanks to the team at RWJF who provided essential leadership and support throughout the development of this manuscript: Ketana Bhavsar, Allyn Brooks-LaSure, Ed Ghisu, and, especially, Kristin Silvani.

Finally, a team of immensely talented writers crafted the manuscript—weaving together multiple narratives, data sources, conference presentations, and extensive interviews into cross-cutting chapters that reflect both the themes of the conference and the subsequent national attention to racial justice and the global pandemic. We are grateful for their rigor, dedication, and creativity. Thank you for your exceptional work, Monica L. Coleman, Karyn Feiden, Mary B. Geisz, Margaret O. Kirk, and Mary Nakashian.

INTRODUCTION

Consider Jackson, Mississippi, in early March 2020. Weeks earlier, record-breaking floods had left the capital's mostly Black residents without safe drinking water for nearly a month. Two weeks later, the city's mayor had declared a civil emergency in response to the appearance of COVID-19. And, in between, the Robert Wood Johnson Foundation (RWJF) held its fifth annual *Sharing Knowledge* conference at the convention center in the heart of downtown.

This volume builds on that conference and then goes much further to reflect the extraordinary events of the period that followed. Our plans to convene, of course, were made with no knowledge of the catastrophic and galvanizing events that were soon to unfold. The location had been chosen instead because we wanted to spotlight the Mississippi capitol, where the influence of systemic racism, past and present, remains on display and where we could reflect on the profound health and racial inequities that result from it. Being in the City with Soul also enabled us to see firsthand the determined struggle of so many residents working to increase justice and equity in their community. We wanted to be in Jackson because we understood it to be a city with stories that have never been fully told, in a state whose flag no longer carriers a Confederate symbol but still houses the Ross Barnett Reservoir, named after a former governor and renowned segregationist.

It was, in short, a setting in which we could build on our conviction that a Culture of Health is impossible without a full-bore commitment to racial equity. For three days, hundreds of conference presenters and participants from around the country engaged in authentic dialogue about the systems and structures that are doing such grave harm to people of color. With so many types of knowledge-builders in the room, a palette of blunt, provocative, and insistent ideas and strategies could be shared to inspire action. Recognizing that the surrounding

Necessary Conversations. Edited by: Alonzo L. Plough, Oxford University Press. © Robert Wood Johnson Foundation 2022.
DOI: 10.1093/oso/9780197641477.001.0001

community had been eyewitness to so much history, we also came together at Two Museums Mississippi, which offers a curated narrative of the state's complex past, and visited the assassination site of activist Medgar Evers and Jackson State University, where the police killings of two Black students in 1970 is now taught as part of the school's orientation program and classroom work.*

The conversations at the conference were edgy, with a sense of urgency that was palpable. Many of our speakers felt that a solutions-focused approach was key—given the well-established influence of the social determinants of health, they wanted to see less focus on continued research of the problem and more on-the-ground work to change narratives, reorient mindsets, and transform policy.

Action-oriented leadership is not a new concept to RWJF, and we have worked to improve health for all since our establishment as a national philanthropy in 1972. Our early work included efforts to increase the representation of people of color in the medical field and to address chronic homelessness and the AIDS epidemic, reduce tobacco use, and reverse the epidemic of childhood obesity. We launched the Culture of Health framework in 2014, calling for all individuals, organizations, communities and sectors to value health as a shared goal, and added health equity to that framework the following year.†

But this book and the *Sharing Knowledge* conference itself reflect a distinct shift in our emphasis that has been emerging in recent years, based on a growing body of evidence that racism is the underlying cause of so many poor health outcomes. By the time we came to Jackson, we had begun to consider what it would take to overhaul institutions that treat people differently on the basis of their race and to make very intentional shifts in our investments to elevate that focus. We had recognized that we had to commit resources and join with others to support working to advance health and racial equity. We had also deepened our understanding of what it means to build partnerships and community power and the centrality of leadership by those who are most affected by the decisions that influence their lives.

We were also keeping a wary eye on a nascent virus. In his *Washington Post* opinion piece as the conference opened, RWJF's President and CEO Richard Besser called out the policy failures that had already intensified health disparities

---

* The terms "people of color" and "communities of color" are used throughout this volume as a broad way to talk about multiple non-White populations, although we recognize there are significant distinctions among subgroups. Some researchers and advocates also use the term Black, Indigenous, and People of Color (BIPOC) to highlight their individuality, but that term is used in this book only where it is part of a quote. Also, note that the terms African American, Black, and Black American are used interchangeably in this volume, as are the terms White and White American. We recognize that language is evolving and that preferences vary.

† Summaries of the Foundation's history and major earlier investments appear in *To Improve Health and Healthcare*, the annual anthology that preceded this *Culture of Health* series.

across the country. With 28 million people lacking health insurance and nearly one-third of the population underinsured, in a country that lacks universal sick leave or family medical leave, and with low-wage and non-salaried workers at highest risk, it was already clear who would be most badly hurt should COVID-19 explode into a full-blown pandemic. "The greatest strains will fall on certain demographics because of their economic, social, or health status," wrote Besser. "And the vulnerabilities will be exposed for all to see during this crisis."[1]

As indeed they were. In the months following the conference, a fissure turned into a chasm as the disease galloped through Black and Brown communities, not because of biology but because of the racism that has shaped the conditions influencing their life course. That pernicious influence, amplified through too many American institutions, revealed power imbalances that sustained inequitable conditions over a long arc of history.

And then came George Floyd's murder in May 2020, every excruciating second captured by Darnella Frazier, a courageous teenager with a cellphone. Police brutality was already well known to communities of color on the afternoon that police officer Derek Chauvin put his knee on Floyd's neck and pinned him against the pavement for 9 minutes and 29 seconds. *Sharing Knowledge* conferences had long included presentations on bias within the criminal justice system and the health harms it inflicts. Yet this event, in all its stark visibility, set a spark. When the video of Floyd ricocheted across social media, followed by an outpouring of enraged and anguished protests, the recognition of racial inequity finally seemed to take hold among a broader audience. As people across the nation saw the brutal realities of racism for themselves, a new narrative, with new goals, began to emerge. Not everyone shed their insistence that the murder represented the work of a few bad actors, rather than a systemic failure, but shifts in the conversation were palpable.

At RWJF, the pandemic and the horror of Floyd's killing warned us to move further, faster in the direction we had already begun. And over the past year, that is what we have done. As we become ever more explicit about the health impacts of structural racism, we have redoubled our efforts to be the kind of partner who listens more closely to those whose lived experience has earned them the trust of their communities and seeks out new grantees, especially among multi-issue, anti-racist groups. We have refined our thinking about how best to catalyze our influence and investments to confront the issues we care about. To drive transformative change, we have brought together funders and researchers in a Health Equity Research Learning Collaborative; supported scholars from diverse, underrepresented, and disadvantaged backgrounds through Health Equity Scholars for Action; and established the National Commission to Transform Public Health Data Systems to reimagine how health data are collected, shared, and used to improve health equity. We are also using our institutional position to encourage other institutions to examine their own practices (These and other initiatives are further described in the Epilogue to this book.)

Health equity remains our operational focus, and generating actionable evidence to improve health equity is the pathway to build a culture of health. There are abundant data clearly showing the influence of racism on health outcomes. However, we still seek a fuller understanding of how to move past simply measuring disparities to a focus on how sustainable changes in structural factors and policy improve the conditions for health equity. Achieving sustainable improvement requires support for thriving communities and local assets that build community power. To learn, we are considering opportunities to transform evaluation and work in new ways with evaluators who are redefining rigor and research methodology (a topic explored further in Chapter 10). As they challenge structural assumptions, our partners are teaching us about the imperative of knowledge equivalence—honoring the many ways of knowing—and demonstrating how data, science, and storytelling can be combined to foster narrative change. They also insist that we pay more attention not only to Black and Latino struggles but to all racial and ethnic groups whose voices are often sidelined, including Asian American, Native Hawaiian, Pacific Islander, and Native American communities. Their too frequent exclusion from research and programming is itself a manifestation of systemic racism.

The contributors to this volume have continued their own journeys in a shifting world since the Jackson conference, and that evolution is reflected here. Their dynamic voices give us the roadmap forward as, together, we tackle the underlying causes of health and racial inequities and craft solutions. We open this book with *Setting the Stage: The History, Struggle, and Strength of Mississippi*, painting a portrait of the state in which we convened, where injustice, struggle, and progress seem endlessly in contention—often mirroring the narrative of the country as a whole. The remainder of the book is organized as follows.

Part I: How Racism Becomes a Structural Problem offers a cohesive framework for recognizing and redressing structural racism. Only by exposing racial hierarchy for what it is—deeply embedded systems and structures that position some people as inherently more valuable than others—can we clear a path for equity. Although the issues are often considered as a Black/White binary, the contributors to these chapters remind us that people of color across racial, ethnic, and gender lines confront bias and struggle for justice. Multidirectional conversations create space to strengthen relationships within and across communities of color even as they challenge White dominance.

Part II: The Harms of Racial Injustice digs into some of the specific realms in which people of color carry the weight of inequity and its accompanying health harms. Data and stories bring comparable revelations: Maternal mortality among Black women far exceeds national norms; people who are, or have been, incarcerated are much more likely to live with chronic health conditions and psychiatric disorders; and immigrants, both those with and without legal papers, endure the damaging consequences of dehumanizing rhetoric and fear. Climate change, too, while affecting a broad swath of the population, has its worst impact on non-White populations. Burdened by the weight of history and present-day narratives that lock in disadvantage, these realities speak to the urgency of dismantling discriminatory systems.

Part III: Strategies to Advance Racial Equity suggests what is possible when we acknowledge and learn from the past, embrace new research and evaluation strategies to measure solutions, elevate the importance of narrative change, and create space for those with lived experiences to drive decision-making. To build the inclusive communities that foster opportunity, we must first understand how historical violence and discriminatory policies have fostered contemporary inequity. Those insights can then inform public policies that are the wellspring of equity, paradigms that acknowledge complexity and the shared understanding that is essential to coalition-building, and civic engagement strategies that encourage voting and census participation.

This book concludes with an *Epilogue: RWJF Looks Toward the Future*, which outlines our continuing commitment at the Foundation to learn from our partners, as well as from our own experiences, about how we can best use our institutional voice to advance health and racial equity.

The events of 2020 were an inflection point in an American journey toward health and racial equity. With its universalist perspective—the recognition that everyone is impacted by an inequitable society and that the work of righting the wrongs must be shouldered by us all—this book extends the powerful call to action that we issued at the conference.[2]

Prologue

Setting the Stage: The History, Struggle, and Strength of Mississippi

Pamela Junior, Executive Director, Two Museums Mississippi

Nsombi Lambright-Haynes, MPPA, Executive Director, One Voice

Ed Sivak, Executive Vice President of Policy and Communications, Hope Enterprise Corporation/HOPE Credit Union (HOPE)

Thea Williams-Black, PhD, Founder and CEO, GEMS: Growing Educational Minds for Success Consulting LLC and Former Dean of Education, Supervision, and Instruction/Professor of Education, Tougaloo College

From racial hierarchies to authentic storytelling, the narrative of Mississippi is one of contrasts that parallel and amplify larger national trends in many ways. To study Mississippi, where RWJF held its fifth annual *Sharing Knowledge* conference in March 2020, is to learn how structural racism was built, venerated, and fiercely defended in the United States to maintain the status quo of non-White disenfranchisement. Yet the story of the state is also one of strength, rooted in a people who have worked collectively and in community to fight a system designed to punch back.

Four Mississippians help to tell that story as they deconstruct historical events, deepen understanding of current issues in the state, and correct the narrative. Uniquely skilled at learning from their struggles, each contributor has taken a different path toward the common goal of dismantling structural racism. Pamela Junior, proud native Mississippian and curator of its history, reflects on a journey that took her from a childhood shaped by school integration struggles to a position as head of one of the largest museums in the state. Ed Sivak, long-time

Pamela Junior, Nsombi Lambright-Haynes, Ed Sivak, and Thea Williams-Black, *Prologue* In: *Necessary Conversations*. Edited by: Alonzo L. Plough, Oxford University Press. © Robert Wood Johnson Foundation 2022. DOI: 10.1093/oso/9780197641477.003.0001

economic justice advocate at Hope Enterprise Corporation/HOPE Credit Union (HOPE), draws a link between structural racism and persistent poverty as he describes transformative community investments. Nsombi Lambright-Haynes, policy advocate and community organizer at One Voice Mississippi, discusses programs empowering individuals and communities across the state. Finally, Thea Williams-Black, education advocate, explores early learning and its impact on the state and its people.

A Persistent Power Struggle

The Choctaws, the Indigenous peoples of what became Mississippi, were the first to face the brutality of White settlers determined to dominate the region. By dint of their resistance and endurance, they also became a model of the indomitable spirit that has made survival possible for so many disenfranchised populations in the state. While many of the Choctaws were violently removed to Oklahoma, one group refused to be forced out by White settlers, and their descendants are today a major presence across 10 counties, contributing significantly to the state's economy.

The Native people who insisted on staying also became allies in the struggle against slavery. The notorious Natchez Indian Revolt of 1729 led to a bloody defeat for the Natchez Indians, who were then forced into slavery themselves.[1] It is not an historical stretch to suggest that subjugation became a motive for them to join forces with others pursuing freedom. That act of coming together to resist White supremacy—the doctrine that assumes the superiority of the White race, whether through conscious belief or the assumption of special privileges—would become something familiar to minority and marginalized groups in the state in the centuries that followed.

Despite that origin story, tensions in Mississippi have long been framed primarily around issues of Black and White. While that is starting to change (see Chapter 2), the demographics of the state lend themselves to dichotomous dialogue—in 2019, Mississippi's population was 59% White, almost 38% Black, 3.4% Latino, 0.6% American Indian and Alaska Native, and 0.1% Native Hawaiian and other Pacific Islander.[2]

Those demographics also help to explain a history that Pamela Junior describes in three words: "Complex. Hard. Romanticized." Junior is a Black woman born in the late 1950s and raised in the state's capitol, barely a mile from Jackson State University, the scene of a violent struggle during the civil rights movements of the 1960s and 1970s. If "romanticized" seems an unlikely part of the description, consider that thousands of visitors from all of the world pour in every year to tour the spectacular antebellum homes of Natchez, about 90 miles southwest of Jackson, seemingly with little thought to the reality that slavery made them possible.[3]

One of the first students to enter an all-White school in Jackson after school integration was mandated by the federal government, Junior has witnessed cycles of progress and brutality in a state whose master narrative depicts Black people as "ignorant" and "lazy." But she has experienced, too, the sweet taste of victory, most recently when the state flag, with its appalling Confederate symbols, came down one last time (see Chapter 8).

Junior has served as executive director at Two Museums Mississippi—the two are the Museum of Mississippi and the Mississippi Civil Rights Museum—since 2019. (She was also the inaugural director for the Mississippi Civil Rights Museum.) More than 450,000 visitors from around the world have wandered through its exhibits and galleries, which showcase some of the most painful and shameful events in the state's history. The museums tell the stories of Mississippi's original inhabitants, the people who were enslaved in the state, and the long and continuing resistance to White supremacy and the structural racism that is their legacy.

> *When the Black Lives Matter protests were held in Jackson, the number of people who came out, even in the midst of COVID, was something that brought tears to my eyes. That's how I feel about Mississippians. Our fight is strong, and it comes from our ancestors.*
>
> —Pamela Junior

All Eyes on Mississippi

Mississippi often makes history, but only part of that history has been fully told. For example, the economic success of cotton, made possible by the labor of enslaved people, is well documented. Less recognized is the risk that emancipation posed to the agrarian economy controlled by White people and the steps they took to protect it. With Blacks in the majority during Reconstruction (the state was then 55% Black[4]), Whites in the state legislature created Black Codes to limit the property Black citizens could own and the jobs they could hold. Black Codes were enforced by an all-White police force, whose members were often Confederate veterans. In many ways, these codes foreshadowed the Jim Crow laws that legalized racial segregation in the country until 1968.[5] Despite being nullified, the influence of these laws and others like them lingers as influences on structural racism.

Centuries later, Mississippi continues to make history, but the present-day story is richer and more complete because it is often told by those who lived through it or studied it closely. In the summer of 2020, news media were on hand to capture the ceremony in which the state flag was finally retired. As the cameras panned to the dignitaries with whom she was standing, Pamela Junior found herself reflecting on her own past. The hatred she experienced during school integration was a deeply embedded memory and she knew, too, that her parents and grandparents had endured that same kind of hatred as the old flag waved on. When that bitter symbol was finally lowered, "that hatred," as she called it, was placed in her arms and she took responsibility for telling the story that led to that moment at Two Museums Mississippi.

> *That was a lot of weight that I carried that day—very scared and anxious.*
> *When I was told where I'd be standing, I knew all eyes would be on me.*
>   —Pamela Junior

Against the backdrop of a dark history shines the bright light held by the next generation, says Junior, who sees the museum's young staff pointing the way to a better future. Together, they are working to connect past to present, illuminate truth, and inspire action toward change. As part of that mission, museum staff regularly visit the sites of some of the state's momentous and sometimes horrific events, including the kidnapping and lynching of Emmett Till after he allegedly offended a White woman. The goal of these experiences is to inform staff so they can speak with knowledge and passion to museum visitors.

Junior hopes that the museum will provide space for honest dialogue about racism within its walls and beyond to help individuals connect more deeply to the need to end racism. Sometimes, just a casual encounter is all that is needed to change how someone thinks, she said, recalling a conversation with a White visitor from a small Mississippi town who asserted, "I don't see color." Junior recognized the comment as a teachable moment and invited the woman to acknowledge her identity as a Black woman, rather than to pretend it wasn't there.

> *If you don't see color, you don't see me. You don't see who I am.*
>   —Pamela Junior

Two Museums Mississippi dives deep into many elements of the state's history, opening opportunities for critical dialogue. One exhibit honors the lives of some 600 people who were lynched while another showcases stories from the Freedom Summer, Freedom Riders, and Freedom Schools, when activists challenged the segregation-riddled norms of the region. Another exhibit offers quotes from heroes both famed and unsung who advanced the cause of racial justice—people like Oseola McCarty, who gained national recognition for helping to educate underserved, college-seeking students, and James Meredith, the first Black student to break the color barrier at the University of Mississippi.

The museum also vividly portrays the story of forced penal labor, the determination of women like Fannie Lou Hamer and June E. Johnson, who worked together tirelessly and under attack to register voters during the civil rights movement, and Mary Harrison Lee, a Filipino civil rights activist renowned for her efforts during the Freedom Rides of 1961. Hamer is also noted for coining the phrase "Mississippi appendectomy," which helped to expose the involuntary sterilization of Black women in the state. These, and others like them, were the backbone of the civil rights movement in Mississippi, says Junior.

Tracing Economic Impact to Slavery

Mississippi's painful history is closely tied to the economic reality of slavery. In the years when slavery flourished, Mississippi was awash in money in the early 19th century. The Mississippi Delta became the richest cotton farming land in the country, bestowing unprecedented wealth on the landowners who controlled the cotton crop.[6] Only by understanding that legacy can we talk about the history of economic development in Mississippi, says Ed Sivak, executive vice president of policy and communications for Hope Enterprise Corporation/ HOPE Credit Union (HOPE).

> *I think the history of economic development in Mississippi really starts by acknowledging that the state was built on a plantation economy.*
>
> —Ed Sivak

For a brief period following the Civil War, the Black population gained the right to vote, state leadership reflected the demographics of the region, and Black farm laborers were able to move up the agricultural ladder.[7] But the promise of emancipation and Reconstruction was short-lived. As Blacks gained power, the Ku Klux Klan and other terrorist groups engaged in violent voter intimidation and White leaders clawed back authority and rewrote the constitution.

The Mississippi Constitution of 1890 governs the state to this day, though it has been heavily amended. The constitution made involuntary servitude legal as punishment for crimes, which paved the way for the brutality of penal labor that continues at the infamous Parchman Farm/Mississippi State Penitentiary and elsewhere. The constitution also legalized segregated schools, one in a series of steps establishing a racial hierarchy in the state.[8]

Segregation really set the state on a path for, frankly, its race to the bottom, given its population.

—Ed Sivak

Economics in Mississippi Today

The structures that support White supremacy remain largely intact and Mississippi is today one of the Blackest[9] and poorest states in the union, its economy built primarily on agriculture and low-wage manufacturing. Nearly 20% of Mississippians lived in poverty in 2019, compared to 12.5% in the nation as a whole.[10] And it is worse in rural parts of the state, where 22% of the population is poor.[11]

Agriculture employs 17% of the state's workforce and is its number one industry, valued at $7.3 billion; top crops include poultry, eggs, soybeans, forestry, cotton, corn, cattle, calves, catfish, hay, and rice.[12] Yet, one in five people and one in four children in the state went hungry in 2020.[13] Fifteen percent of the state's population received federal Supplemental Nutrition Assistance Program (SNAP) benefits in 2019[14] and Mississippi is projected to be the most food-insecure state in the union post-COVID.[15]

The degree of segregation is evident in the stark contrasts between counties that share borders. Tunica and DeSoto Counties, for example, are neighboring counties in the northwest corner but have little in common beyond that. According to 2019 census data, Tunica was 78% Black and 20% White, with a median household income of $39,000, while DeSoto, with a population that was 30% Black and 66% White, had a median income of $67,000. More residents of Tunica were poor (28%) compared to DeSoto (9%) and fewer graduated high school (83% compared to 90%). Local tax base differences reflect the "economic segregation" of the counties, skimping on students in low-income areas while giving students in the neighboring district what they need for a quality education.[16]

Defining Persistent Poverty

Half of Mississippi's 82 counties have been designated counties of *persistent poverty*. A technical term used by the federal government to classify counties where poverty rates have remained at 20% or more for the past 30 years, persistent poverty can be found in 407 counties across the nation.[17] More than 10% of those counties are in Mississippi. Decaying infrastructure, schools with leaky roofs, and rural hospitals that have closed down are all signs of persistent poverty, explained HOPE's Ed Sivak.

More than half the residents of Mississippi's counties of persistent poverty are people of color, many with health indicators of deep concern, according to County Health Ranking data published by the Robert Wood Johnson Foundation. Most counties in the bottom quartile of the worst health outcomes are predominantly Black while most in the top quartile are predominantly White.

Two other neighboring counties reveal what that means for health disparities.[18] As of 2021, Lafayette County, which is 70% White and ranked second in the state for health outcomes, has one primary care physician for every 1,600 residents and one mental health provider for every 160 residents. Next door, Panola, whose population is 50% Black, ranks 52nd in health outcomes. That county has one primary care physician for every 4,900 residents and one mental health provider for every 1,000 residents. The data on obesity and longevity are equally stark. In Lafayette, one-third of the population is obese and the average lifespan is 78 years (74 for Blacks and 79 for Whites). In Panola, 44% of the population is obese and the average life expectancy is 73 (72 for Blacks and 73 for Whites).

> *This isn't an accident. This persistent poverty was by design, through policy choices that were put into place to facilitate White supremacy.*
>
> —Ed Sivak

As a part of his role at HOPE, Sivak serves as a member of the Persistent Poverty Working Group, a national coalition that tries to attract public, private, and philanthropic investments into affected areas. In 2016, the coalition secured $401 million from a federal rural lending program designed to support the development of essential community facilities like hospitals, childcare centers, and community gardens; HOPE received $90 million of the funding.[19]

From Transactions to Transformation

HOPE is a Black- and women-owned, Black-led community development financial institution (CDFI) and credit union based in Mississippi that serves "low-wealth people and communities." CDFIs are financial institutions whose primary goals are to provide access to financial services and expand economic opportunities in underserved communities.[20] Launched in 1995 as Mississippi's only church-sponsored credit union at Anderson United Methodist Church in Jackson, HOPE now has 35,000 members and serves individuals throughout Mississippi and surrounding states.[21] Credit unions are not-for-profit financial institutions owned and controlled by the members they serve; their profits are generally used to help members access products and services with low-cost fees, lower interest rates on loans, and higher interest rates on savings accounts.[22]

To meet the needs of marginalized communities in Mississippi and sur-rounding states, HOPE invests in places and projects that other financial institutions would not consider. Since 1994, HOPE has generated more than $2.9 billion in financing that has benefited more than 1.7 million people in Alabama, Arkansas, Louisiana, Mississippi, and Tennessee.[23]

HOPE's success can be credited to its commitment to provide transforma-tive economic development opportunities that go beyond profit-oriented and short-term transactions, Sivak explained. Five years ago in the Mississippi Delta, HOPE took over four traditional bank branches in three counties that were being closed by another financial institution. Prior to reopening the branches, the CEO of HOPE met with local people in those communities to ask a simple question—what do you need?—and then responded by expanding services. Whereas the previous institution only cashed checks and accepted deposits, the branches are now part of the credit union and offer a full suite of financial serv-ices, mortgages, small business loans, car loans, an ATM, and financial educa-tion. In three of the four communities, HOPE is the only financial institution in operation.

The Hope Community Partnership has been central to the organization's suc-cess. Through the program, HOPE supports the convening of local residents to surface key community development priorities. Once identified, HOPE works alongside leaders to import the financial resources needed to bring these projects to fruition. The partnership has been instrumental in securing funding for several smaller projects, including updating a youth baseball field, sponsoring murals, and installing decorative lights from the highway to the center of town. It has also played a critical role in a number of larger projects, such as the re-development of the Eastmoor Subdivision, a community on the outskirts of Moorhead, Miss., that had endured fires, sewage issues, and other substandard living conditions due to neglect by its landlords.[24]

HOPE's innovations have not gone unnoticed. Goldman Sachs recently partnered with HOPE to connect small businesses to the federal Small Business Administration Paycheck Protection Program as part of the economic response to the COVID-19 pandemic. As a result, HOPE was able to make more than 2,600 small business commercial loans in 2020, compared to an average of 40 to 50 in previous years. This program has since concluded. Overall, 89% of the businesses assisted through the program were Black-owned, with a median loan size of $14,063. Sixty-eight percent of loans were to sole proprietors.

Other corporations are also investing heavily in HOPE, including Netflix, which made a $10 million "Transformational Deposit" as part of its commit-ment to racial equity, creating a substantial pool of low-cost funds in the credit union to lend out.[25] "The Transformational Deposit Program allows us to import wealth into places where resources are scarce to expand impact and access to capital," explained Sivak. "It reduces our cost of funds as well, which positions the credit union to invest more efficiently and directly into communities."

HOPE is also working to help rural hospitals access financing. Given the disproportionate number of rural hospital closures in the South and the refusal of many southern states to expand Medicaid, Sivak urged that policy discussions be broadened to encompass the overall rural health infrastructure. "This is where the policy conversation really matters," he said. In addition to resources for rural hospitals, financial support for federally qualified health centers, which are frequently critical sources of both primary care and jobs, has been identified as an essential priority.

Building Power Through Coalitions

Nsombi Lambright-Haynes was born in Mississippi and has lived there most of her life. In her work as executive director of One Voice, she leads several programs designed to empower residents and ensure that the voices of those who have been disenfranchised get heard.

One Voice is a nonprofit organization that was birthed out of the Mississippi State Conference NAACP to advocate for policies that support marginalized communities in the wake of Hurricanes Katrina, Rita, and Wilma in 2005. One Voice continues to work closely with the NAACP, leveraging its membership base to build coalitions. Its approach to developing a progressive civil infrastructure is three-pronged: community organizing, leadership development, and policy reform.

Community Organizing

Mississippi has a long tradition of hospitality, which is all about gathering and welcoming people. One Voice leverages that spirit of "coming together" by focusing on coalition building in local communities, statewide, and with national partners. One state-level coalition is currently focused on civic engagement and others focus on education. Meetings typically involve diverse groups of people discussing issues and developing problem-solving strategies. "Most of our groups do tend to be led by people of color, mostly Black people, but we work with everyone who aligns with our principles," explained Lambright-Haynes. "It really takes a multicultural coalition. Several statewide groups are led by White people who have come to the table, and we also work with some Latinx groups."

Building coalitions in one of the most segregated states in the country is not an easy feat. Lambright-Haynes's bold strategy—convening people who often have conflicting values—adds an extra layer of complexity, but it may also offer the best possibility for progress. For example, One Voice brought together religious leaders, transgender groups, and people who had been formerly incarcerated to advocate for early voting, no-excuse absentee voting, online voter registration, and full restoration of voting rights to individuals with felony convictions. Given the diverse values held by these participants, Lambright-Haynes encourages them to identify and acknowledge their biases and then set them aside in service to collective aims. Although a small number of people have opted out of these eclectic groups, most have been able to recognize the value of accepting differences to pursue common goals.

Allies in Mississippi share One Voice's conviction that coming together is the path forward. One example was the response to the massive statewide Immigration and Customs Enforcement (ICE) raid in 2019, the largest ever to take place at a workplace site, when religious leaders in Black communities joined immigrant groups to denounce the raids. The Mississippi Poor People's Campaign, launched by Martin Luther King Jr. in late 1967, is also a showcase for the power of multicultural coalitions. Today, the campaign is a national movement that rallies working families to fight "the evils of systemic racism, poverty, the war economy, ecological devastation and the nation's distorted morality of religious nationalism."[26]

Leadership Institutes

The Mississippi Black Leadership Institute is a One Voice forum that convenes state leaders in a series of nine monthly meetings to share strategies for recognizing and dismantling structural racism. During their time together, participants also work on a community transformation project that focuses on equity. Often these projects endure, as with Six Dimensions LLC, a national public health consulting firm designed to bring awareness to Black maternal health (see Chapter 4). Nakeitra Burse, DrPh, CHES, established Six Dimensions in 2017 when she was at the leadership institute.[27]

Now in its 10th class, the institute also helps to prepare leaders for political office, creating a diverse pipeline of qualified candidates, which has the potential to shift political power in the state. Several of its alumni currently serve in the Mississippi House of Representatives, while others are district attorneys, county attorneys, county supervisors, and entrepreneurs.

Current events often influence the conversations at the monthly meetings and provide a forum to link issues in Mississippi with those elsewhere in the nation. For example, the group read *The New Jim Crow* by Michelle Alexander, about the nation's shameful mass incarceration policies, and then discussed the criminal justice system in Mississippi. That, in turn, evolved into a broader conversation about police brutality in the state and nationwide.

Another One Voice initiative, the Electric Cooperative Leadership Institute, aims to address imbalances within the state's electrical cooperatives. Many Mississippi residents purchase their power through such co-ops, which were created in the 1930s with federal loans to help bring electricity to rural areas. Residents who get their power through these co-ops are member-owners who elect a board of directors; each co-op board then elects its own officers and hires a general manager.

The Electric Cooperative Leadership Institute was established because consumers were not always aware of their member-owner status, what that means, or their right to vote and participate in annual meetings—something One Voice discovered while researching ways to help residents who were complaining of high electric bills. Ultimately, its goal is to diversify the boards, but this has been a challenge, with co-op boards remaining mostly White, even where the community is predominantly Black. Without intending the double entendre, Lambright-Haynes calls that gap a "power struggle." More successful have been efforts to teach member-owners how to access funding from the co-op to improve their communities and to educate them about the local impacts of climate justice.

Representation and Policy Reform

Lack of representation is not limited to electric co-ops—it is also an issue in state leadership and a potent barrier to statewide policy reform. While Black candidates have taken seats in local elections, they often struggle to win statewide offices. Voting patterns suggest this is at least partly because many White people will vote only for other Whites, regardless of party affiliation.

"Party demographics suggest that if most African Americans vote Democrat—and they vote along with White Democrats in Mississippi—we should be able to get a Black person elected," asserted Lambright-Haynes. Despite the obvious bias indicated by the failure to do so, she is optimistic that organizations like hers can diminish the power of oppressive structures in the state. The change in the state flag suggests that is possible.

> *Years and years of organizing work finally bubbled up to systemic statewide reform, and I think we can do a lot more.*
>
> —Nsombi Lambright-Haynes

Ultimately, Lambright-Haynes says, progress begins with empathy. "We have to really see ourselves in this work. As an educated Black woman, I have to really see myself in the sister around the corner who is receiving pandemic benefits and maybe unemployment benefits. We are impacted by the same system. And so if I don't see myself in that family, then I'm missing part of the importance of this work."

Creating Change Through Education

As a former dean of education at Tougaloo College, the oldest teacher education program in Mississippi, Thea Williams-Black has long "seen herself in the work." Her expertise centers on the importance of engaging children early in the learning process and elevating the role that higher education plays in preparing teachers. As an educational leader, Williams-Black's professional journey afforded her opportunities across the country, but ultimately she returned to her alma mater to teach and lead.

"I felt like I needed to go back because Tougaloo is where teacher education started in the state of Mississippi, especially for African Americans," she said.

The Role of Early Education

Williams-Black is from a family that has long influenced education in the state. In the late 1970s, Mississippi was one of only two states that did not fund kindergarten programs (North Dakota was the other).[28] When he was a gubernatorial candidate, William Winter called for a pilot kindergarten program, and after his victory, Williams-Black's mother took a leading role in helping to pilot the initiative. Statewide kindergarten programs were established in 1982.

Williams-Black is proud that Mississippi now offers kindergarten, although enrollment is not required. She sees a direct connection between opportunities to improve access to the program and racial achievement gaps in the state, noting that low-income families are particularly disenfranchised if they cannot send their children to kindergarten.

As a child, she had access and support to educational resources and knows from research that family involvement motivates students to engage in learning and reading.[29] Yet she is well aware that many parents, especially in poor households, face barriers to becoming involved in their children's education. In one family, where a child was being raised by a grandparent, the adult praised the child for reading a book but did not move past praise to find out whether the child actually understood the content. An important component of kindergarten programs is their family engagement strategies, which can include home visits, information and services to promote understanding of child development, and opportunities to involve families in learning activities.[30]

> *All students do have parents who want them to excel. They just don't know what to do to help them to excel.*
>
> —Thea Williams-Black

One of the key roles of kindergarten is to help students with "learning to learn," including the basic vocabulary, language, and math skills they need to do well in first grade. Research indicates that most children who come from impoverished homes have limited vocabulary and that by age 5 their scores on standardized tests that measure language development show them to be an average of two years behind their age group.[31] Early learning programs can help address that gap.

Mississippi's Kindergarten Readiness Assessment program, which has benchmarks at the beginning and end of the year, demonstrates the potential. Students are expected to enter kindergarten able to identity most of the alphabet, match letters to sounds, and read picture books and familiar words. By the end of the year, they should have mastered alphabet skills and letter/sound relationships and be able to identify some consonant and vowel sounds; blend sounds and word parts; read simple words; and use pictures, story patterns, and phonics to figure out words.[32] In research examining the school years 2017–18 and 2018–19, most students in the state (64%) entered the program below the benchmark but 62% to 65% were able to get on track by the end of the year.[33,34] Williams-Black sees this evidence of kindergarten's effectiveness at preparing students for first grade as a powerful argument for mandating it for all children.

> *We're expecting our students to be able to read when they leave kindergarten based on these state tests, but kindergarten is not mandated.*
>
> —Thea Williams-Black

Preparing 21st-Century Teachers

Along with elevating the importance of kindergarten and family involvement in education, Williams-Black recognizes the need to link research and practice to grow teachers ready to meet the demands of the 21st century. That requires preparing teachers to do things a little differently than they have been done in the past—something her students are not always quick to accept.

In Mississippi, restructuring educational systems is rarely easy to do. Teaching is a poorly rewarded profession in the state, with salaries starting below $40,000 for first-year teachers. Some aspiring teachers are themselves from impoverished backgrounds, lack broad life experiences, and may be the first generation in their family to attend college. Many also need remedial skills training, as suggested in their scores on the Praxis Core Academic Skills for Educators (Praxis I), which is commonly used in teacher preparation programs to assess reading, writing, and math abilities.

In addition to offering tutoring and other academic supports at Tougaloo, Williams-Black encourages her students to dive into research and present their work at conferences and other scholarly events, a strategy she hopes will open their minds and lead to a shift in the culture of teaching practices statewide. "Times have changed," she said, describing the message she tries to convey. "That is not to mock your teacher who taught for 40 some years but to let you know 'this is what the researchers are saying, and this is how we should go about doing it.'"

> *Nothing's wrong with how your teacher did it, but this is how we're going to do it moving forward.*
>
> —Thea Williams-Black

Williams-Black uses several research-based strategies to prepare students to teach in diverse settings. She emphasizes teaching soft skills, such as how to communicate professionally; connects learning to educational standards; encourages students to pursue their own research opportunities; and offers a "model classroom" that nurtures critical thinking while showing students how to arrange a classroom and teach content. Group work is also emphasized, given that the professional world increasingly relies on teams that require students to "think outside the box."

Looking to educators like William-Black as sources of inspiration, Mississippi teachers show a determination that belies their limited resources and is too often underappreciated. In the Delta region, for example, some schools have found innovative ways to thrive in the virtual learning environment engendered by the pandemic, using Google Slides, Google Classroom, Zoom, and breakout sessions. Yet this work has not gained the attention it deserves, nor has it been positioned as a potential model for others, says Williams-Black. "No one's even looking at them because they're small, and they're low performing," she commented, explaining how places with a reputation for underperforming are not expected to develop exemplars considered worth replicating.

Perhaps the most challenging issue in the state's efforts to expand early education and 21st-century learning is one that also plagues the nation—a shortage of teachers of color. Only 21% of the workforce within Mississippi's school system are Black women (Black males represent just 6%),[35] yet Black students make up almost half the public school population. Teachers who complete the Tougaloo program can help fill the gap, but it will take innovation, commitment, and resources to guide them there.

The Final Word

Despite the many deep and committed efforts to advancing racial equity and a multitude of other social justice causes in Mississippi, the myth persists that residents are all too willing to accept the chronic poverty and economic, education, and health disparities that haunt the state. That is not so, but Mississippians have rarely been given time to tell their own stories or to recognize the significance of their own achievements. Having struggled against so much for so long—and along the way seen remarkable victories, crushing defeats, and a long path ahead—they have tended to downplay all of what they have accomplished.

> *That's what African Americans do. And you don't realize that what you're doing is a great thing because we've had to do it for so long. You just did what you had to do.*
>
> —Thea Williams-Black

Though it comes slowly, progress in the state is on the horizon. As the nation embraces its long journey toward racial reconciliation, Mississippi may have the furthest to go and the most to gain. Signs that the state is ready for the work are everywhere. The diverse audiences that flock to Two Museums Mississippi are making room for a collective focus on racial healing through art and storytelling, painful though it is. Corporate citizens and nonprofit organizations like HOPE are supporting business and financial innovations, targeting areas plagued by chronic poverty and bridging historical capital gaps. As One Voice continues to develop a pipeline of leaders working to dismantle structural racism in their local communities, the first college for teachers in the state is readying the next generation of educators who will advance literacy and drive educational achievement.

Mississippi is on the move. It must be, lest its people get left behind.

PART I

HOW RACISM BECOMES A STRUCTURAL PROBLEM

The United States is at a moment of reckoning with our past and present on matters of race. To move forward, we will need to fully understand our history and come to terms with the ways in which it still shapes and sustains present-day institutions, policies, and practices that hold us back from achieving health equity. Structural racism refers to the persistence of inequity in communities of color, with other Americans benefiting from a disproportionate share of the nation's resources. The impacts of this inequity are cross-generational and include lack of basic healthcare, education, housing, and other essentials. A deep and collective reckoning is essential if a healthier and more equitable future is to be possible for all.

The three chapters in this opening section frame the ways in which structural racism persists and influences directly unfair health outcomes in communities of color across the nation. This is in spite of decades of public policies and community action to mitigate this influence. By linking historical events with current circumstances, the contributors provide a broad backdrop for future action. They are a diverse group—advocates, community representatives, journalists, and academics—and they illustrate how a pervasive system of racial hierarchy, widespread "othering" of groups and individuals, and the inability to hold authentic conversations undermine health and equity. Yet hope remains a source of inspiration for all of them as they lay out pathways to change.

In Chapter 1, "Racial Hierarchy, Race Narrative, and the Structures That Sustain Them," a leader in health and healing, a Pulitzer Prize–winning journalist, and the president of a national civil rights organization paint a comprehensive picture of how racism becomes a structural problem for our country. Exposing the racial hierarchy that has shaped the United States, the narratives that ignore the unavoidable consequences of enslavement in our history and our present, and the structural racism that endures, they also propose alternatives to promote racial healing and transformation, restore wealth to Black Americans, and create anti-racist institutions.

In Chapter 2, "Beyond the Black/White Binary: Confronting Invisibility and the Harms of 'Othering,'" four contributors—one White, one Latino, one Indigenous, and one transgender—reflect on the commonalities that characterize many historically disenfranchised populations and their too-frequent omission from conversations about race. Observations from leaders of Asian descent create a fuller picture of the populations who are too often left out of research, programming, and policy. Together, they illustrate the harms caused when some groups remain invisible and highlight the opportunities to improve everyone's well-being by standing together on common ground.

The part concludes with Chapter 3, "Keeping It Real: Pathways to Authentic Connections." Reflections from five contributors capture a powerful recurring theme of the *Sharing Knowledge* conference: Authentic conversations are essential, difficult, and urgent. Embedded racial hierarchy and the pervasive "othering" of many populations prevent people from talking honestly about racism. Without fully embracing the discomfort of our collective history with race, conversation and narratives often generate unproductive fear, shame, guilt, avoidance, and denial. Using examples from their work, the contributors suggest ways to overcome obstacles. Nonetheless, the request from one contributor to remain anonymous out of fear of reprisal is a sobering reminder that much work remains.

Racial Hierarchy, Race Narrative, and the Structures That Sustain Them

Gail C. Christopher, DN, Executive Director, National Collaborative for Health Equity (NCHE); Founder of Ntianu Garden: Center for Healing and Nature; Senior Scholar, Center for the Advancement of Well-Being, George Mason University

Nikole Hannah-Jones, MA, Domestic correspondent, the New York Times

Derrick Johnson, JD, President and Chief Executive Officer, NAACP

Prevailing narratives about the United States often paint a rosy picture of steady progress toward freedom and equity. Fewer narratives address the nation's darker story in which access to basic healthcare and a decent education, safety from violence, and the right to participate in civic society are unavailable to many. Civil rights legislation that outlaws specific discriminatory behaviors, while an essential step forward, has neither ensured equity nor overturned underlying structural racism.

Too many people continue to be denied opportunities to benefit from the social and economic wealth they helped to create. Early settlers and their descendants engaged in deliberate and brutal oppression of Native Americans, denying them their land and outlawing their cultures. African Americans, whose ancestors were kidnapped by profiteers and forced onto slave ships, are still burdened by policies that first solidified their status as property and later codified them as second-class citizens. Asian Americans live with the legacy of the 1882 Chinese Exclusion Act, which suspended Chinese immigration and prohibited Chinese people living here from applying for citizenship, and memories that Japanese Americans were interred in their own country during World War II. Immigrants from a variety of other countries continue to confront a wall of

Gail C.Christopher, Nikole Hannah-Jones, and Derrick Johnson, *Racial Hierarchy, Race Narrative, and the Structures That Sustain Them* In: *Necessary Conversations*. Edited by: Alonzo L. Plough, Oxford University Press. © Robert Wood Johnson Foundation 2022. DOI: 10.1093/oso/9780197641477.003.0002

structural obstacles that block their efforts to earn a living, attend school, or be full members of the society in which they live.

RWJF president and CEO Richard Besser put the problem directly to *Sharing Knowledge* conference participants:

> In our country, there are people who have a lifetime of benefits and opportunities starting at birth because that's how we've structured our society. Others face a stack of barriers and burdens that have nothing to do with how hard they work or how much education they have, because society has set it up that way. And if this inequity is to improve, we have to recognize it, we have to call it out, and we have to work to change it.

The contributors to this chapter build on Besser's call to action with complementary perspectives on racism and inequity. From different angles, they come to a shared conviction that meaningful change is imperative and urgent.

The chapter opens with Gail Christopher's discussion of the racial hierarchy of human value that spawns profound racial injustice, and her thoughts on how to achieve racial truth, healing, and transformation. Nikole Hannah-Jones then challenges predominant narratives about race. Her Pulitzer Prize–winning *1619 Project*, which exposes the legacy of slavery, and her call for reparations aim to reframe the ways in which people understand oppression and its effects, even as she remains dubious about the prospect for real progress. Derrick Johnson concludes the chapter by examining how institutions and power imbalances sustain racial injustice, using examples from history and observations from current events.

A Racial Hierarchy of Human Value

After struggling through her own childhood health challenges and coming to terms with the premature death of her infant daughter, whose condition was neglected by the medical system, Gail Christopher has dedicated her life to the principle that all people matter. Trained as a doctor of naprapathic medicine, a holistic health profession that uses manual musculoskeletal manipulations and nutritional, lifestyle, and behavioral counseling to relieve pain and to promote health and well-being, she has been a leader in the fields of family preservation and government innovation and a senior philanthropist. She currently serves as executive director of the National Collaborative for Health Equity.

A central theme of Christopher's work has been exposing, explaining, and eliminating the racial hierarchy that has plagued the United States since its inception. At its core, racial hierarchy assigns different value to different groups— value being a measure of who and what society believes to matter. While this hierarchy undermines everyone's well-being and freedom, Black people, Latino people and other people of color are most affected. The decimation of Indigenous people, the enslavement of Black people, the stereotyped biases against Asian Americans, and the harsh approach to immigrants have endured for centuries because American institutions have been constructed to devalue them.*

> *If you live in the United States you have been part of a cultural dynamic that adheres to the fallacy that some human beings have more value than others based on how they look.*
>
> —Gail Christopher

Only by jettisoning racial hierarchy, Christopher believes, can we heal our bodies, minds, and spirits. "In order to move forward, this nation must heal the wounds of our past and learn to work together with civility, and indeed, with love," she said. "We must build the capacity to see ourselves in the face of the other."

The Roots and Reach of Racial Hierarchy

Racial hierarchy has deep historical roots, many grounded in falsehoods that have operated under the guise of science. In 1758, Swedish botanist Carolus Linnaeus (dubbed the father of modern taxonomy) added physical and moral attributes to his 1735 taxonomy of human beings. "The result of this expansion of the classification of man was the 10th edition of *systema naturae*, which became the basis for scientific racism," according to the Linnaean Society of London.[1]

Linnaeus described four human species along five attributes: skin color, body posture, and medical temperament (based on ancient humoral theory that the interaction of four bodily fluids—blood, yellow bile, phlegm, and black bile—explains differences in disposition)[2]; physical traits relating to hair, eyes, and face; behavior; manner of clothing; and form of government. Descriptions from a classification table are paraphrased below:

- *Americanus* species are unyielding, cheerful, and free. Members are governed by customary right. They have straight, black, and thick hair; gaping nostrils; freckled faces; and beardless chins. Their coloring and body type are red, choleric, and straight.

---

* Sources differ as to the use of the term *Latino* or the gender-neutral *Latinx* as a descriptor for all members of that community. Inevitably, this leads to a degree of inconsistency, but in this volume, *Latino* is generally used to refer to the entire population while *Latina* is used only where the female gender is specified. *Latinx* is used when the term is used in quoted material or a data source.

- *Europaeus* species are light, wise, and inventive. They are governed by rites. Members have yellow hair and blue eyes. Their coloring and body type are white, sanguine, and muscular.
- *Asiaticus* species are stern, haughty, and greedy. They are governed by opinions. Their coloring and body type are sallow, melancholic, and stiff. They have blackish hair and dark eyes.
- *Africanus* species are sly, sluggish, and neglectful. They are governed by caprice. Their coloring and body type are Black, phlegmatic, and lazy. Members have dark hair, with many twisting braids; silky skin; flat nose; swollen lips; women with elongated labia; breasts lactating profusely.

Linnaeus's taxonomy was widely accepted by scientists and philosophers and shaped popular opinion for centuries.

Also during this period, White colonists in the nascent United States were uniting around a desire for freedom and economic security, with some convinced that was possible only by continuing to enslave Black people. The country's framing principles solidified racial hierarchy by positioning Black people as unworthy of freedom and legitimizing the rights of Whites to own them.

Myths about biological inferiority endured, but by the end of the 20th century, scientific advances published by the International Human Genome Sequencing Consortium had thoroughly debunked beliefs that races differ in their physiological makeup and character. More than 2,800 researchers shared authorship of the publication,[3] which appeared in *Nature* in 2001.[4] The National Human Genome Center, a unit within the National Institutes of Health (NIH), reports, "Though these visible traits [skin color and facial features] are influenced by genes, the vast majority of genetic variation exists within racial groups and not between them. Race is an ideology and for this reason, many scientists believe that race should be more accurately described as a social construct and not a biological one."[5]

With that history as backdrop, and always motivated by her understanding that American institutions and traditions continue to reinforce a hierarchy of value framed by race, Christopher developed an agenda for moving the needle toward racial justice and equity.

Harnessing the Human Spirit for Positive Change

Christopher believes in the power of the human spirit to forge an equitable society. "Our hearts and brains are designed to resonate with harmonious relationships," she said. "The opposite—fear and anxiety, separation, alienation, and hate—induces stress and distress, which causes a cascade of illness in our physical bodies and our body politic."

Taking her cue from visionary R. Buckminster Fuller, who believed that systems don't change by arguing against reality but rather by offering a new model that makes the existing one obsolete, Christopher is dedicated to offering a new model.

> *I prefer to talk about what I am for than about what I am against, and in race, we haven't focused a lot on what we are for.*
>
> —Gail Christopher

Two incidents on the same wrenching day in May 2020 showcase entrenched racial bias yet also promise a glimmer of hope that new models can emerge. First, the shocking killing of George Floyd, a Black man, by a White police officer in Minneapolis prompted a groundswell of outrage across the country. "George Floyd cried for his mother. Everyone has a mother," Christopher said. "That cry allowed each of us to see ourselves in Mr. Floyd's face."

More than a thousand miles away, Amy Cooper, a White woman, was walking her dog off-leash in a section of New York's Central Park favored by birdwatchers where leashes are required. When George Cooper (no relation), a Black birdwatcher, asked Ms. Cooper to leash her dog, she called 911 instead, her voice rising frantically as she claimed that "an African American man" was threatening her. Her baseless accusations, too, were captured on video in real time.

These events, coming shortly after the February murder of Ahmaud Arbery in Georgia, the March murder of Breonna Taylor in Kentucky, and other attacks on unarmed Black people, shocked the nation and indeed the world, and people of all ages and races poured onto the streets—setting aside their fears during a pandemic—to join in calls for reform. They also spurred policymakers to reflect not only on the abhorrent behavior of a few individuals but also on the underlying models that enable such behaviors.

"People's biases emerge in times of stress and their perceived options become more narrow," observed Christopher. "And that is why it is so dangerous for a police officer, surgeon, classroom teacher, or immigration officer to harbor deep-seated biases and lack policy protections that prevent their biases from shaping the lives of others." It is time, she added, for all of us to take responsibility for the harm caused by bias and work together for change.

Creating Equitable Institutions, Changing Hearts and Minds

Academics and activists frequently debate whether removing racist structures or working to change hearts and minds is a more effective strategy. Christopher considers this a false dichotomy, asserting, "Our nation does not have the luxury of getting bogged down in it."

Equitable policies and institutions are essential, she agrees, but will endure only if they are backed by strong beliefs. She argues, "Changing structures might work for an election cycle or even a generation, but that change is only temporary if it sits on top of the same undergirding frame that some people have less value than others."

"People were demonstrating on behalf of George Floyd because their hearts had been affected," she noted. "But we need to have an intentional development of skills around empathy and compassion and human understanding. We need to learn those skills just like we learned how to read."

Christopher's "Truth, Racial Healing, and Transformation" framework aims to provide those skills by guiding people in joining together in the work of changing hearts, minds, and institutions (see the Spotlight in the next chapter, which describes a core component of this framework).

The framework gained traction in 2020 when Representative Barbara Lee (D-Calif.) and Senator Cory Booker (D-N.J.) introduced a concurrent resolution proposing a "U.S. Commission on Truth, Racial Healing, and Transformation to properly acknowledge, memorialize, and be a catalyst for progress, including toward permanently eliminating persistent racial inequities.[6]

Ultimately, Christopher concludes, a spiritual belief system is the guiding force. "I honestly feel that most people are basically good at heart, and we have to create spaces for that goodness to be expressed," she emphasizes. "It's not that I'm not angry. I am angry. But I've learned to channel that anger to bring about positive change. I don't want the only Black person that most Whites see to be George Floyd being killed by a police officer."

A Story That Needs to Be Told

New York Times journalist Nikole Hannah-Jones creates powerful and provocative narratives to enlighten, engage, and push for change. Her inaugural article, written for her high school newspaper, described her experiences as a Black child being bused to a White school. "I think what drives my work is telling the story that I think needs to be told," she said, "and if I tell it in a compelling way, in an evocative way, and in a way that can be backed up by fact, hopefully I will draw some other people in."

> *Narrative matters because it is the lens through which we understand facts and the way we interpret them.*
>
> —Nikole Hannah-Jones

Hannah-Jones's work challenges prevailing narratives about the founding of the United States, which largely overlook or misrepresent centuries of brutal oppression of Black Americans. "The United States is a nation founded on both an ideal and a lie," she contends, noting that its principles of " 'life, liberty, and the pursuit of happiness' did not apply to fully one-fifth of the country"[7] when they appeared in the Declaration of Independence.

The embedded narrative further suggests that the United States has moved steadily along a path toward progress since achieving independence. Hannah-Jones does not accept that. In reality, a racial caste system hardened after the country won its independence, backed by laws constraining the rights of Black Americans and scientific papers asserting that Black people were not fully human. "The Supreme Court enshrined this thinking in its 1857 Dred Scott decision," she wrote, "ruling that Black people, whether enslaved or free, came from a 'slave' race." This decision, she said, "became the root of the endemic racism that we still cannot purge from this nation today."[8]

Since the enactment of civil rights legislation, the American narrative has evolved to peg the unequal status of Black people either to their own personal failures or to racist views held by a limited number of individuals. "That is not how this has ever worked," Hannah-Jones said. "There is a structure and an architecture that created inequality, and those exist whether individuals operate with racial animus or not."

Hannah-Jones's analyses and writings about segregation, racism, and injustice have earned her multiple accolades, including a MacArthur Fellowship and a Pulitzer Prize. In August 2019, the *New York Times Magazine* devoted an entire issue to her landmark 1619 Project, which challenges everyone to come to terms with the full history of both the ideal and the lie of the United States.

The 1619 Project: A Different Narrative of American History

Launched exactly 400 years after the first enslaved Africans reached American shores, the 1619 Project "aims to reframe the country's history by placing the consequences of slavery and the contributions of Black Americans at the very center of our national narrative,"[9] reads the *New York Times* announcement of the project.

> *This project is really trying to reframe, in the American mind, no matter what the politics of that person are, the way that we have been taught to think about our country.*
>
> —Nikole Hannah-Jones

Hannah-Jones directs the project, which launched with essays and commentaries challenging common understanding about enslavement, the contributions of enslaved people in building the American economy and democracy, and the legacy of slavery. Written by experts in history, healthcare, music, and other fields, the breadth and tone of the essays are suggested by some of their titles:

- "In Order to Understand the Brutality of American Capitalism, You Have to Start on the Plantation" (Matthew Desmond)
- "A Traffic Jam in Atlanta Would Seem to Have Nothing to Do with Slavery. But Look Closer . . ." (Kevin M. Kruse)
- "Myths About Physical Racial Differences Were Used to Justify Slavery— And Are Still Believed by Doctors Today" (Linda Villarosa) (see Chapter 4 for more on Villarosa's work)
- "For Centuries, Black Music, Forged in Bondage, Has Been the Sound of Complete Artistic Freedom. No Wonder Everybody Is Always Stealing it." (Wesley Morris)

As a continuing initiative, the 1619 Project features a podcast series as well as a school curriculum with supporting material curated by the Pulitzer Center, a Washington-based nonprofit dedicated to supporting quality journalism examining underreported issues.

The 1619 Project generated immediate and explosive responses—a 2020 Pulitzer Prize for Hannah-Jones, rave reviews, allegations of inaccuracy, and a call to rescind the Pulitzer. These responses reflected "how unsettling this project is," said Hannah-Jones, and indicate "the reach it is having outside of the people who we would normally think would engage with a project like this."

Hannah-Jones leverages her outrage to reach people and engage them in action: "What I find useful is a sense of rage over the choices we make every day that some people are valuable, and some people aren't. I don't want us to feel hopeful that we will change it one day. I want us to do something about it right now."

> Across our country, across racial demographics, across class, there is a profound misunderstanding of the role that racism, racial caste plays in our society, in how foundational slavery is.
>
> —Nikole Hannah-Jones

Controversies over the project escalated in 2021, when some states introduced bills to cut funding to schools and colleges that teach the 1619 Project curriculum.[10] In June, the Florida Board of Education adopted a rule that would ban public schools from using it in the classroom.[11]

Narratives That Mislead: Anti-Black Racism in Health and Education

Focusing through the RWJF lens of a Culture of Health, Hannah-Jones reflected on the ways segregation and racism affect two foundational markers of well-being: health and education. Segregation, she said, has been more than a means of demeaning Black citizens and denying them their basic rights. Rather, it enables "opportunity hoarding," by physically isolating Black Americans from opportunities while allowing Whites disproportionate access to them.

> *Segregation was a means of preventing Black people from having access to services that White Americans enjoyed in order to keep Black people on the bottom of the racial caste system and to ensure that White Americans remained on top.*
>
> —Nikole Hannah-Jones

Public education, for example, is considered "a great equalizer," Hannah-Jones notes, yet curricula gloss over nearly 250 years of enslavement and 100 more years of state-sanctioned oppression. Today, segregation functions to ensure that Black and Latino children attend schools that deprive them of access to the best instruction, healthy learning environments, and even basic resources such as textbooks.

The current emphasis on charter schools as the vehicle to improve education drains resources out of public systems and diminishes the democracy of elected school boards in Black and low-income communities, said Hannah-Jones: "Let us be clear: Charter schools do not go into wealthy White communities. They go into either racially diverse communities as a tool of segregation, or they go into completely segregated Black and Brown communities as providing a so-called option."

Likewise with health. The racism baked into the country's DNA, Hannah-Jones believes, created systems that once made it permissible to sell Black children because they allowed White Americans to believe that enslaved mothers couldn't possibly love their offspring in the same way that Whites do. The wellspring of those beliefs endures in the kinds of assumptions that allow healthcare providers to act as if Black people feel pain differently.

Today, White Americans are less likely to support social programs if they believe large numbers of Black people will benefit from them, Hannah-Jones said. Mississippi, for example, refuses to expand Medicaid to low-income families, many of whom are White, because Black families will disproportionately benefit from the expansion program, she added. (See the Prologue for more about the conference host state.)

"It is important in narrative to tie these fates together," noted Hannah-Jones, in order to make clear that the harms of anti-Black racism are not limited to Black communities, and that Whites, too, suffer when racism is allowed to persist. "The coronavirus," she suggested, "is exposing that we are all connected and that our desire to deny something to people we think are undeserving could actually hurt all of us."

What Is Owed: Reparations

Hannah-Jones seized on the outcry after George Floyd's murder to talk about the debts owed to Black descendants of enslaved people. While protests alone don't create justice, she perceived in the marches a willingness to consider more fundamental changes.

> If we are truly at the precipice of a transformative moment, the most tragic of outcomes would be that the demand be too timid and the resolution too small.
>
> —Nikole Hannah-Jones[12]

"What Is Owed," Hannah-Jones's article calling for reparations, appeared in the *New York Times Magazine* in late June 2020. "None of the actions we are told Black people must take if they want to 'lift themselves' out of poverty and gain financial stability—not marrying, not getting educated, not saving more, not owning a home—can mitigate 400 years of racialized plundering,"[13] she wrote.

Wealth—assets and investments minus debt—is a significant indicator of well-being and one denied to most Black people since the time they were kidnapped from Africa. Closing the wealth gap should be the guiding principle for reparations, Hannah-Jones asserted.

> While unchecked discrimination still plays a significant role in shunting opportunities for Black Americans, it is White Americans' centuries-long economic head start that most effectively maintains racial caste today.— Nikole Hannah-Jones[14]

The frame through which to view reparations is that they are the responsibility of all Americans, not only those whose ancestors were slave owners. They are not a tool for punishing White people, Hannah-Jones said, but rather an obligation of a nation that sanctioned enslavement from its inception, continued to protect it, and practiced legal segregation and discrimination until half a century ago.

Reparations, she believes, should be available to "any person who has documentation that he or she identified as a Black person for at least 10 years before the beginning of any reparations process and can trace at least one ancestor back to American slavery."[15] Along with individual cash payments to descendants of those who had been enslaved, reparations must include commitments to enforcing existing prohibitions against discrimination and targeted investments in segregated Black communities and schools.[16]

The technical components are the easier part, however. The real obstacle, Hannah-Jones said, is convincing enough people that the centuries of forced economic oppression should be remedied, "that restitution is owed to people who have never had an equal chance to take advantage of the bounty they played such a significant part in creating."[17]

Power for People

Giving people that equal chance is core to the mission of the NAACP, a catalyst and leader in promoting racial justice, health, and equity for more than 110 years and widely considered one of the most far-reaching civil rights organizations in the United States and beyond.

Derrick Johnson, NAACP's president and CEO, directs the work of more than half a million members, 2,200 branch or unit offices, and 2 million volunteers across the country.[18] Johnson joined the NAACP as a volunteer in 1990 and has served as president of both the Tougaloo College and Mississippi state chapter, and later as a national board member. Having seen the organization from many angles over the decades, he is now committed to building on its legacy to "reimagine our posture looking forward to 2030 or 2040." Johnson evokes the image of the mythological African Sankofa—a bird in flight, pushing forward while its head looks back—to illustrate his vision.

Structure, Not Mindset

Johnson's dual training as an activist and an attorney has shaped his belief that governance is about power, which he defines as the capacity to either make things happen or to impede them. Rather than dwelling on the racist beliefs of individuals, he sees the real counterweight to racism as equitable structures and systems, leading him to focus more on changing institutions rather than beliefs.

> *It's about structure. While individual mindsets influence structure, for long-term systemic change to take place, there must also be a focus on institutions and structures.*
>
> —Derrick Johnson

Pundits and the media can appeal to people's hearts, Johnson acknowledged. "But if a child is being denied quality education because of his or her ZIP code, that's not about a heart, that's about deliberate and intentional structural racism." He offers two examples from history and one from the present day to illustrate what happens when policies fail to address embedded racism.

New Deal Initiatives

President Franklin D. Roosevelt's New Deal initiatives were acclaimed for enhancing the role of the federal government in leveling the economic playing field. In failing to address the racist underpinnings of the institutions responsible for administering those initiatives, however, New Deal benefits were not made available to many Black and low-income people. For example, domestic and agricultural jobs, traditionally major sources of employment for Black Americans, were not covered by Social Security, leaving these long-time workers impoverished in their later years of life.

A particularly notorious example of structural racism was the home mortgage guarantee administered by the Federal Housing Administration (FHA), which was steered to White buyers. FHA explicitly included guidance that preference be given to people and areas with safeguards to prevent "the infiltration of . . . lower class occupancy and inharmonious racial groups."[19] This and tactics such as redlining—the discriminatory practice of denying loans and other resources to residents of certain areas—were further impediments to homeownership that have to this day denied Black people access to a significant source of intergenerational wealth. (See Chapter 8 for more on how past policies influence home ownership and residential segregation to this day, and Chapter 9 to reflect on practices being used to create affordable housing and drive more equitable communities.)

Education Policies

The history of education also illustrates how a racist infrastructure endures over time, despite allegedly race-neutral or progressive policies, Johnson said, seconding arguments made by Hannah-Jones. Enslaved children were prohibited from attending school, and when Black schools did open after the Civil War, policies were enacted to steer public resources to Whites-only schools.

When the Supreme Court ordered public schools to be desegregated "with all deliberate speed" in its landmark 1954 decision *Brown v. Board of Education of Topeka,* forceful and sometimes violent protests ensued, including attempts to physically block Black children from entering school buildings. Some jurisdictions closed public schools entirely, offering tuition benefits for children to attend private schools that had Whites-only policies in place.[20]

More than 65 years later, school segregation remains pervasive and many of the underlying mechanisms that allow it to continue are still intact. Indeed, there have been steps backwards, including the Supreme Court's 1974 *Milliken v. Bradley* ruling that school district lines do not have to be redrawn to promote desegregation, unless deliberately discriminatory acts have occurred.[21]

The result: In 2017, Black children were five times as likely as White children to attend highly segregated schools, according to the Economic Policy Institute.[22] And a 2019 *New York Times* article reported, "At Stuyvesant High School [a highly selective public high school in New York City], out of 895 slots in the freshman class, only seven were offered to Black students," down from only 10 in the prior year and 13 the year before that.[23]

Primary reliance on local property taxes to fund schools is one of the fundamental structural impediments to opportunity within low-income communities. As the *New York Times* reported, "School districts that predominantly serve students of color received $23 billion less in funding than mostly White school districts in the United States in 2016, despite serving the same number of students.[24]

Contemporary debates about charter schools distract attention from the historical failure to invest in educating Black and low-income children, Johnson said. That failure allowed those schools to "run into the ground so that private charter school vendors can enter education and profit from it, without accountability," he asserted. Black and low-income families face the choice of sending their children to poorly performing public schools or to charter schools, "and neither of them has done us a service," he noted.

When COVID-19 Became a Black Disease

As an example of the structural inequities that cry out for broad-based change, COVID-19 is as timely as can be. Early in the pandemic, Johnson hoped that the country might enter a period of shared unity to defeat the disease. Surely, he thought, the most serious threat to the physical and economic health of the country in a century would encourage us to rally together in common cause.

That hope didn't last. "From embracing stay-at-home orders . . . we've come to see armed protestors storm state capitols to end the lockdown," Johnson wrote in a May 11, 2020, CNN blog.[25]

For a minute there, it looked like we were all in this together. And then we weren't.

—Derrick Johnson

What changed? Johnson's answer: "The face of the pandemic changed. It became Black." In early April, a month after the pandemic began to escalate, the Centers for Disease Control and Prevention (CDC) reported that while Black people represented 13% of the U.S. population, they represented 33% of patients hospitalized for COVID-19.[26] Conversely, Latino people represented 18% of the population but just 8% of those who were hospitalized.[27] With that, Johnson concluded, "the fragile sense of social solidarity that was keeping millions of Americans at home to protect each other began to crumble."[28]

Black people are especially vulnerable because they make up a disproportionate share of the essential workers who are most likely to be infected by the virus. They are also more likely to live in crowded housing and environmentally toxic neighborhoods, making them more vulnerable to acute illness and death.

Johnson urges us not to allow the COVID-19 crisis to become another instance of "White flight," this time from the realities of health inequity. Instead, he writes, "We could answer the call to rise together and fight the pandemic, using science and reason as our guides and democracy as our beacon. Our nation's fractured history does not need to be our destiny."[29]

Democracy and the Power of the Vote

Success depends in no small part on a fair voting system. Johnson believes that is fundamental to addressing racist structures because voters elect the officials who will determine policy and tax decisions. Equitable tax policies, in turn, shore up democracy by blunting the distortion of resources that ensues when rampant capitalism is left unchecked. By contrast, when democracy is weak, "people get exploited, systems get altered, and resources get pillaged."

Since taking the helm at the NAACP in 2017, Johnson has been implementing a five-year plan to build the organization's technology, legal, and communications infrastructure on behalf of promoting fair elections and civic engagement. That infrastructure proved to be a critical resource through the 2020 presidential campaign and election. "We [the NAACP] are nonpartisan," Johnson noted. "We don't tell people how to vote; we just want to make sure their voices are part of the conversation."

Informed by data generated by a research and analytics firm, the NAACP targeted select states and communities. One project, for example, aimed to increase voting among registered African Americans with spotty voting records by 5% to 7%, the level needed to affect local outcomes in the area. Another matched local NAACP volunteers with neighborhood residents. Initially envisioned as a boots-on-the-ground, get-out-the-vote initiative, the work pivoted to mail, telephone, and online outreach after COVID-19 precluded most direct personal contact.

"At the same time, we aggressively monitored the electoral processes and filed lawsuits to be sure votes were not stolen," Johnson said. "We have people on the ground in every community, so we have standing to file lawsuits anywhere and to become strong plaintiffs." (See Chapter 11 for more about voting.)

A Final Word

As they follow their different paths toward racial justice and equity, each of the contributors to this chapter points the way forward. Gail Christopher's context-setting framework, Nikole Hannah-Jones's incisive narrative, and Derrick Johnson's insights into power offer a richer understanding of America's sins, past and present, and the opportunities to redress them.

"Citizens don't inherit just the glory of their nation, but its wrongs too," said Nikole Hannah-Jones, concluding her call for reparations. "A truly great country does not ignore or excuse its sins. It confronts them and then works to make them right."[30] Perhaps that work has begun. In March 2021, the city of Evanston, Illinois, issued $25,000 grants toward home purchases or repairs to qualifying Black residents, the first phase of its 10-year commitment to distribute $10 million in reparations.[31]

As we move through the third decade of the 20th century, the country is at an inflection point, believes Johnson. The national outcry after the George Floyd murder brought together grieving, determined, and angry people across lines: "It is Blacks, it's Whites, it's males, it's females, young and old, and they are all rallying behind the value proposition that Black lives matter. And the value proposition is one of empathy and inclusion. And it shows the solidarity around what is possible."

> *That is the place where we are as a nation, whether we will work towards a different future or allow the gravitational pull of the past. How do we make democracy work for everyone?*
>
> —Derrick Johnson

Beyond the Black/White Binary

Confronting Invisibility and the Harms of "Othering"

Juan Cartagena, President and General Counsel, LatinoJustice

Shelby Chestnut, MS, Director of Policy and Programs, Transgender Law Center

Crystal Echo Hawk, MA, Executive Director, IllumiNative

Donna Ladd, Founding Editor, Mississippi Free Press and Jackson Free Press

"Damn it, we're a little complicated." With his slightly tongue-in-cheek remark, Juan Cartagena described the diversity of Latino communities and warned against making sweeping generalizations about any group. Americans, he suggests, can be sorted not only by country of origin, but by political outlook, views on authority and criminal justice, reasons for coming to the United States, and the influences all of that has on first-generation immigrants and the generations that follow.

The complications of American society do not, of course, stop there. This chapter brings together four contributors who go beyond the Black/White binary so often used to talk about people of color, a reference point that at once leaves out many other populations who share American soil and overlooks the threads that tie them together. The stories recounted here tell of poor White people who learn almost from birth to "other" Black people, blaming them for anything wrong with their lives; of the many immigrant groups who once hailed from the Spanish-speaking countries to the south; of Native Americans whose ancestry long predates the first colonists; of Asian Americans who are so often left out of research, policies, and programs that target non-White communities; and of transgender people, especially from communities of color.

Juan Cartagena, Shelby Chestnut, Crystal Echo Hawk, and Donna Ladd, *Beyond the Black/White Binary* In: *Necessary Conversations*. Edited by: Alonzo L. Plough, Oxford University Press. © Robert Wood Johnson Foundation 2022. DOI: 10.1093/oso/9780197641477.003.0003

The whole country is complex and becoming increasingly more so.
—Juan Cartagena

As it highlights the distinctiveness of these subpopulations, the chapter also plants the seeds for solidarity. Like African Americans, these groups have been shuttered from many of the opportunities conferred on privileged Whites and often made to feel invisible and somehow "less than." They, too, have been pegged as having lesser value, reflecting the racial hierarchy explored in Chapter 1. This provides an opportunity to examine similarities among people who have faced injustice and the tensions that sometimes obscure their common ground. Building alliances that can level the playing field, promote self-determination, and build power requires understanding the characteristics, complexities, and nuances within and across diverse populations.

Donna Ladd's worldview is reflected in the *Jackson Free Press*, the award-winning news weekly she founded in 2002, and the newer statewide, nonprofit publication *Mississippi Free Press*, both of which probe structural racism like no other Mississippi media outlet. Launched to provide in-depth reporting across historical divides, to introduce members of different communities to one another, and especially to help educate White people about the Black experience, the publications' coverage also includes in-depth pieces about immigrants, the LGBTQ community, and the Choctaws, who first lived on the land that is now Mississippi.

As he paints a fuller portrait of Latino people, Juan Cartagena also spotlights the legacy of dominance that has denigrated the community's unique cultural contributions, blurred knowledge of its richness through faulty data collection, and sometimes generated internal tensions. But he offers hope, too, that by "decolonizing the mind," Latino people can claim their rightful presence on the American landscape.

Crystal Echo Hawk speaks of "a master narrative, a narrative that has not been authored by Native peoples up until now" and explains why that needs to change. She presents startling data about how little Americans know about Indigenous people and their rich culture, which has endured despite the anguish of displacement and genocide. The challenges facing people of Asian descent—often overlooked amidst stereotypes of a monolithic "model minority"—are examined in this chapter as well. Finally, Shelby Chestnut describes the transgender community's push to influence or lead the research, philanthropy, and policy that affects them. Welcoming the opportunity to present at the *Sharing Knowledge* conference, Chestnut commented, "As a queer, Indigenous trans person who's a community organizer, I don't oftentimes get invited to spaces like this."

The Power of Othering

A White woman, Donna Ladd was raised in Mississippi poverty, where norms encouraged Whites, whatever their economic status, to feel superior to Black people. "We were supposed to blame everybody else for our own problems," she recalled. "There was so much fear-mongering about the 'other.'"

> *You don't want to be on the bottom rung of the ladder so you grab on to any implication that you are not the worst, no matter what we might have in common.*
>
> —Donna Ladd

In the closed, racist culture in which she lived, her mother, who learned to read only in her 60s, worked in a factory side by side with Black and Choctaw people and developed a level of empathy that was rare to her time and place. Ladd attributes her own early awakening on racial justice to her compassionate mother, teachers who took her under their wings, and the shocking moment of awareness when she learned at the age of 14 that three civil rights workers, James Cheney, Andrew Goodman, and Michael Schwerner, had been murdered in her hometown of Philadelphia, Mississippi.

A deeper understanding came as she dug into history. In a life characterized by cultural humility, Ladd learned to listen deeply and realized, "I wasn't looking closely enough at Whiteness. I was dancing around it." Lectures and conversations with Black intellectuals at the Columbia University School of Journalism in New York City sharpened her awareness of the realities of Black lives and the misconceptions perpetuated by the media and other institutions, she said. In Dr. Manning Marable's class on Black intellectualism, Ladd rarely spoke, instead seeking out "remarkable people who had things to teach me. I listened and I did the reading and had conversations with people who had things to tell me or corrected me."

All of that opened her eyes to a broader context. By positioning Black people as "others" to be blamed and feared, Ladd understood that it was possible for White people and the institutions they control to keep their systems of privilege in place. "The powerful are the people who benefit the most from racism throughout our history as a nation," she emphasized. "They have done everything they can to dehumanize Black people in the eyes of those who can help support a system of White supremacy."

Her lifelong journey to educate herself continues, Ladd said: "I have spent my whole life trying to learn what I wasn't taught growing up as a White person in Mississippi."

Cutting-Edge Journalism in Mississippi

At the *Jackson Free Press*, and the newer *Mississippi Free Press*, which Ladd co-founded in March 2020 to extend similar cutting-edge journalism to the entire state, Black issues remain front and center, but broadened coverage has become a priority. "I don't want binary thinking," she explained. "One of the biggest problems is that society forces us into comparisons—'well, at least that is better than this.'"

A shoestring operation when it launched, the *Jackson Free Press* was welcomed enthusiastically in Black areas of the city—but startled some of its readers with a story entitled "Men We Love" that featured a White gay man and his husband. "We love what you are doing with the paper, but we don't know about this gay stuff," said a proprietor of a Black-owned barber and beauty shop quizzically to Ladd.

Thus began a conversation in which Ladd talked about the role she saw for the *Jackson Free Press*. "I said something along the lines of 'at the very core of our mission is this idea that all of our people, all Jacksonians have value.' People are treated very poorly in the Black community and in other marginalized groups. Part of what we represent is this idea of what we all have in common."

Ladd's goals for expanding coverage statewide build on the recognition that a Black/White framework does not produce a full portrait of Mississippi and that the true history of the state has rarely been told. The exclusion of the Choctaws—not only in media, but also in mainstream education and popular narrative—is a particularly notable omission (see the Prologue to this book). The first inhabitants of the southeastern United States, these Indigenous people retain tribal membership, but their history and culture is barely acknowledged in Mississippi. "From the very beginning our state was created by stealing land from Native Americans. No one is learning the history of these people," declared Ladd. "We were raised with such blind ignorance and miseducation about other people. That is White supremacy."

> *In Mississippi, everything is Black and White so often. We haven't done a great job in our state widening that conversation.*
>
> —Donna Ladd

Incorporating other stories into the narrative sweep of racial injustice is as vital as it is nuanced and needs to be done without "lessening the need to really examine the Black/White dynamic and the miseducation that is keeping that hierarchy in place," Ladd argued. Billboarding the strengths of so many American communities, rather than highlighting their deficits, is one humanizing tool in the hands of media. "There are not enough stories about who we are, our hopes, our dreams, our successes," one Latina journalist told her.

With the *Jackson Free Press* playing a prominent role in fostering dialogue and introducing low-resource communities to one another, alliances have been built in Mississippi that Ladd believes would not once have been possible. Black Mississippians have stood up for LGBTQ people, the LGBTQ community has reached out to diversify its ranks, and connections have been forged among various immigrant groups. "Truth-telling and deep listening and then empathy are very important," said Ladd. "Giving people space to come along can be really important. But that doesn't mean holding back information that might challenge their beliefs."

By becoming more inclusive in its coverage, the media can become a player in breaking down false narratives and dissolving stereotypes. "Media has a special role because we have been guilty throughout U.S. history—both implicitly and explicitly—about who we covered and how we cover them," she acknowledged. "People need to see themselves represented in the media. If we don't do that we are solidifying the divisions and the hierarchy about who deserves coverage, whose stories deserve to be told."

The Latino Experience

In the more urban Northeast, Juan Cartagena's very different childhood led him to many of the same conclusions about the power of "othering" and the dangers of division. A Puerto Rican man raised by a single mother in a racially mixed Jersey City, New Jersey, neighborhood, Cartagena says his upbringing was "the perfect way to understand that Puerto Rican struggles, Latino struggles, are the same as African American struggles in many ways, shapes, and forms."

It also gave him a lens through which to view economic injustice. From the moment he earned his first paycheck as a public interest attorney, reflecting a salary that was substantially larger than that of his mother, who had worked 30 years as a sewing machine operator, Cartagena says that economic injustice gnawed at him. "I couldn't believe how this country values, or actually misvalues, the people who work with their hands, the people who make this country what it is," he lamented.

Advocating for investments that level the playing field of opportunity is a central focus of Cartagena's leadership role at LatinoJustice, a civil rights law firm that champions criminal justice, economic justice, immigrant rights, voting rights, human rights for Puerto Rico, and other issues of central importance to the Latino community.

From Different to Dehumanized

Understanding the "complications" of the Latino population, which numbers some 60 million in the United States, begins with glimpsing its diversity in the United States. Two-thirds of the people in that broad category hail originally from Mexico and 16% come from Puerto Rico, with Salvadorans and Cubans as the next two largest groups. All of their stories are unique, both within and across national boundaries. Puerto Ricans are, of course, U.S. citizens while other Latino people have legal status as citizens or residents, live here without documentation, or are part of mixed-status families. Some have been here for decades or longer; others migrated much more recently, motivated by the political situation in their home countries, safety fears, the desire to pursue educational or economic opportunities, or the yearning to join family.

Many research designs fail to capture these variations. While clinical investigations—such as studies of vaccine efficacy or the prevalence of a health condition—have evolved to capture race and ethnicity reasonably well, data collection in areas such as criminal justice, education, and infrastructure has not. That oversight has numerous implications for policy and advocacy. Many states, for example, cannot provide the most basic information about arrests, probation, parole, or incarceration among the Latino population as a whole, let alone make distinctions within it. Instead, they obscure the realities of those who interface with the criminal justice system by labeling them Black, White, or "other."

The consequences became apparent to a young man named Angel Sánchez who starred in a LatinoJustice videotape highlighting the Latino data gap. Now a University of Miami law student, Sánchez spent 12 years in prison, where officials insisted on labeling him as White. He kept saying, "No, I'm Latino," an insistence that became a test of wills, leading prison officials to threaten him with isolation. After his release, Sánchez dug deeper into the faulty recordkeeping of the Florida Department of Corrections and now studies ways to use other databases to correct them (watch "Decolonize Justice: Latino Data Gap" to learn more[1]).

Sanchez's prison experience, said Cartagena, "is a stark reminder that sometimes we let systems tell us or determine what our race and ethnicity is," an approach that defies Census Bureau best practices for allowing individuals to choose their own identity (see Chapter 11). It also becomes a tool for rendering populations invisible—if their existence is barely acknowledged, their contributions are easily overlooked. "That creates a sense of 'othering,' of seeing these communities as 'less than,'" Cartagena warned.

The result is what he calls the "criminalization of presence," even among communities that have been home to generations of Latino populations. Angel Mercedez, a high school student and artist who spoke at the *Sharing Knowledge* conference, explained what that looks like in a young person's life. Fluent in

English, spoken with a Spanish accent, he has been routinely asked "Are you Mexican?" and "Are you here legally?" since arriving in the United States from the Dominican Republic.

"It's the predetermined thought from children who grow up in the same community as me and learn through the same systems of education to immediately assume that their classmate is here illegally and for the wrong reasons," Mercedez observed.

Othering is a convenient strategy for dehumanizing an entire community. In a society that perceives White norms as the standard of proper behavior, any deviation becomes suspect. Injunctions against gang affiliations that are enforced only for Latino young men and public school policies that impose racially biased dress codes and rules governing hairstyles[2] are examples of the consequences. "Many youths my age in the Latinx community suffer from being forced to keep their cultural norms within a small group of people, not expressing their viewpoints, their thoughts, perhaps their music, dance and food," said Mercedez. "And this creates a lack of openness which then creates mistrust."

Divisions from Within

Pressures on the Latino community come not only from external forces but sometimes also from within the community itself, a reminder that othering has a power that defies logic. It is a testament, too, to Gail Christopher's observation that to live in the United States is to internalize racial hierarchy (see Chapter 1).

A national poll conducted by LatinoJustice, for example, asked Latino people what they thought should be done to reduce crime. Funding rehabilitation programs was the overwhelming choice, outpolling three others (deportation, more money for police, and more money for prisons) by a 2:1 ratio. But 12% of the respondents favored deportation as a pathway to crime prevention.[3] In reality, according to the National Academy of Sciences, undocumented immigrants are *half as likely* to be arrested as U.S.-born citizens,[4] but this evidence that has not been enough to dispel false narratives.

Attitudes toward legal status have too often become a source of rupture within the Latino community. "It is not uncommon for immigrants of any race or national origin to start developing notions about newcomers," said Cartagena, suggesting they sometimes view immigration as a zero–sum game: "There is a pattern that says, 'I got here, my grandkids are fine, maybe we should close the door on immigrants.' Our legal status in this country can be a breaking point."

The wellspring of that division traces far back into history, he explained. Most enslaved Africans were taken first to the Caribbean or to Central and South America, where skin color and other physiological features eventually reflected the blending of Black, European, and Indigenous cultures. As their descendants migrated to the United States, many carried with them a preference for lighter skin, echoing the racial sensibilities that were already well established here.

"Colorism," a hierarchy within racial groups that privileges paler complexions, has been one expression of this experience. Cartagena calls it "an assault on blackness . . . a tendency to value appearances, to assume intelligence or dominance or appropriateness based on people's skin color." As a child, he heard jokes about *pelo bueno* and *pelo malo*, good hair and bad hair, just one example of ingrained racism. Without full awareness, the Latino community has latched onto the biases of White culture, a dynamic captured by a Pew Research Center study finding that "Hispanics with darker skin are more likely to experience discrimination than those with lighter skin."[5]

> *There is a level of privilege that attaches to whiteness. And not just whiteness writ large, but also colorism.*
>
> —Juan Cartagena

Confronting that kind of White dominance begins with a process of "decolonization," Cartagena said. Colonization—which he defines as the domination and subjugation of peoples deemed less worthy—has been a driving force in American society for so long that it often goes unrecognized. For marginalized people to claim their rightful place, he said, "We have to decolonize our bodies, our minds, our neighborhoods, our communities. Our presence in this country needs to be exalted and elevated by way of addressing this notion of dominance."

Unpacking the dynamics of power and privilege leads quickly to the intersection at which so many marginalized populations meet. "You have to understand how this country created policies, laws, and practices to make life impossible for people of Asian American, Native American, and Latin ancestry," explained Cartagena, taking history as his guide. "We have to fully understand the Chinese Exclusion Act [late-19th-century legislation that excluded all Chinese immigrants] and Operation Wetback [a mid-20th-century government initiative], which repatriated almost a million Mexican-Americans through federal edict."

The intent is not to compare relative deprivation and discrimination, but to agree on root causes. "It is not that we are saying 'we suffered, too'—that's not it at all. It is to say we need a better understanding of why we are in this place and to understand the history and policies that have made wealth easier to accumulate for some groups than others."

"We don't do things in isolation," Cartagena concluded. "We have to recognize that in order to change the dial and create more investment in our communities, we have to fight against anti-Blackness. We have to make sure that it's front and center of what we do. We have to fight against any kind of exclusion of people because of their gender preferences."

> Recognize that what we're doing here is tied at the hip to what's happening to people of color throughout the country. Anchor it in the intersectionality of our approaches.
>
> —Juan Cartagena

Like Donna Ladd, Cartagena recognizes the imperative of asset-based storytelling. "Let's talk about the stories of the family members who are making a decent living and opening up a small business and what that means for the kids, what it means for them as they are becoming self-sustaining members of their own community," he urged. "What does it mean about their faith, what does it mean about how they're proud of being a part of society and how they're proud that they finally made it here and what does it mean for their grandkids? Those are the kinds of stories we need."

Reclaiming Native Truth

The anti-Black sentiment that Ladd describes and the invisibility that Cartagena associates with the failure to collect Latino-specific data return as themes in exploring the status of Indigenous people. Discrepancies in the population count of the Choctaw nation are but a single example of the shaky foundation on which policies are too often based and resources allocated: Differences in data sources led the U.S. Census to recognize only 24,000 members of the present-day Choctaw Nation, while the tribe's own rolls include 200,000 members.[6]

Wells of Ignorance

To dig deeper into the deficits of knowledge about Indigenous populations that course through American institutions, Crystal Echo Hawk, executive director of the Native people's advocacy group IllumiNative, co-led Reclaiming Native Truth, the largest-ever public opinion research project about Native peoples.[7] Funded with a $3.2 million investment from the W.K. Kellogg Foundation, its goal, she said, was to "uncover the national conversation about Native peoples . . . to get into the minds of Americans and into influential institutions in America that have the greatest impact on Native peoples in order to understand their master narratives. What do people think they know about us and why is that? How do these perceptions begin to manifest and affect us at all levels of society?"

To answer those questions, researchers undertook a comprehensive literature review; held 28 focus groups in 10 states; surveyed 13,000 people; conducted 45 in-depth interviews with leaders in government, entertainment, philanthropy, and other sectors; analyzed some 45 million social media posts; and more. The overarching finding: Invisibility is the biggest barrier faced by Native people.

> *The power of invisibility is that it serves to dehumanize. Invisibility is the modern form of racism against Native peoples.*
>
> —Crystal Echo Hawk

Another powerful research takeaway is that systems, not individuals, are the force perpetuating the erasure of Native peoples from public awareness. As the 2018 project report states, "Across the education curriculum, pop culture entertainment, news media, social media, and the judicial system, the voices and stories of contemporary Native peoples are missing. Into this void springs an antiquated or romanticized narrative, ripe with myths and misperceptions."

Among many other eye-openers, the study highlighted a finding from earlier research showing that nearly 87% of schools in this country teach nothing about Native peoples after 1900.[8] Likewise, 95% of the images that turn up in a search of the term "Native American" on the Google images database have 19th-century origins. Native people are hidden by the media as well, representing less than 0.04% of television and film characters.[9] When they do appear, characters are variously depicted as savage, mystical, alcoholic, or oversexualized and the storylines in which they are featured are again well over a century old.[10]

All of that contributes to stunning ignorance—78% of Americans say they know little to nothing about Native people.[11] The reality that tribal nations have the political status of sovereign nations recognized within the Constitution of the United States is overlooked. The values of spirituality, commitment to family, connection to art and culture, and the sense of environmental responsibility that are at the heart of Native American life are unacknowledged. "We're really relegated to being like ancient civilizations," said Echo Hawk, who is often asked whether she lives in a teepee. "Generation after generation of American children are coming through our institutions and being conditioned to think we no longer exist."

Without facts, fiction takes center stage, allowing caricatures of the Native population to gain broad acceptance. Until the summer of 2020, the football stadium of the Kansas City Chiefs was often filled to overflowing with fans in redface and ceremonial headdresses. "If there was a stadium of people in blackface, we would never have stood for that," Echo Hawk said. "Yet it is somehow institutionalized in the country that it is okay to have this level of racism on display about Native peoples."

Although the Chiefs finally barred fans from arriving in headdresses and redface, the team has not changed its name, nor have the Buffalo Bills, the Atlanta Braves, the Florida State Seminoles, or the Fighting Illini at the University of Illinois, among many others. These demeaning monikers do documented harm, as do the Tomahawk Chop, war chants, redface, and feathered clothing, which remain commonplace in sports venues. One scholarly research review called out a broad set of damaging effects from the use of Native American mascots, finding that they foster low self-esteem and other negative psychosocial outcomes, fuel stereotypes and prejudice, and undermine intergroup relations.[12]

"It's not okay to get up and play Indian because it doesn't honor Native people, it harms us," asserted Echo Hawk. "And the science is there. This is not about being politically correct, it is about protecting the well-being of Native American children and Native peoples."

Just as Cartagena recognized that colorism divides people within the Latino community and Ladd saw how some Whites buy into the myth that Black people are the cause of their marginalization, Echo Hawk acknowledged the wedge that sometimes comes between Native Americans and other communities of color. One claim that surfaced repeatedly in the *Reclaiming Native Truth* research is that Native people receive more than their fair share of government benefits and cash payments. "I heard they get checks for every child they have," alleged one Black focus group participant.

That kind of falsehood not only exposes widespread lack of knowledge about the history of tribal treaties and the promises made in exchange for Indigenous land, but also illustrates the insidious ways in which the "master narrative" of White supremacy surfaces. "We have to understand the role of narrative in culture and societies and how much it consciously and unconsciously shapes how we show up, how we act in the world, how structures and systems are," insisted Echo Hawk.

"There are a lot of core narratives that keep us separate from one another," she explained, noting the frames perpetuated by White-dominated systems of media, government, education, and culture. "When we should be finding ways to come together, these great myths, these kind of dominant narratives about one another, sow division instead."

> *White supremacy is one of our greatest evils. We need to look at that and how*
> *it shows up in our communities in the way that we're looking at each other.*
> —Crystal Echo Hawk

As the Black Lives Matter movement gained momentum in the summer of 2020, it brought the issue of systematic racism to the fore, said Echo Hawk, but it needs to go further. "We need to talk about everyone at every level. That is the importance of the movement that erupted. That is where we need to go. You have to look at the way Black people are treated, but you also need to say what the experience of Indigenous people is. It is *both/and.*"

Misconceptions About Asian Americans

Americans of Asian descent face a comparable struggle to call attention to the realities of their lives. "Where are you from?" is a question too often asked of Asian American and Pacific Islander (AAPI) people whose families have been in this country for generations, a microaggression revealing that we remain a society that still considers White skin the norm.

Much else about the community is poorly understood as well, as a package of rigorous data assembled as part of a National Public Radio project reveals.[13] Some of the ignorance is the result of research methodology that groups all people of Asian descent together, masking significant differences by country of origin. This aggregation of data masks significant social and health differences— for example, 70% of Asian Indian adults have a college degree, compared with only 26% of Vietnamese adults. Likewise, more than 35% of the Korean population in New York City are smokers, compared to only 14.1% of all Asians.[14] (See the Epilogue in this book to learn about the Transforming Public Health Data Systems to Advance Health Equity initiative and its advocacy for data disaggregation.)

One result is to feed misconceptions about income and educational levels, immigration patterns, and the degree to which the AAPI people have been subject to discrimination and structural racism. The history of violence targeted at these populations over the centuries are little known. Yet from laws that prohibited Asian Americans from testifying against White people in California, to massacres in Los Angeles and Wyoming and Ku Klux Klan attacks in Texas, to the Chinese Exclusion Act and the Japanese internment camps, the Asian experience on U.S. soil has rarely been smooth.[15]

> *While the bigoted rhetoric about COVID-19 may have exacerbated hate against Asian Americans, it has been with us for generations.*
>
> —RWJF blog[16]

During the COVID-19 pandemic, ignorance and vitriol combined to allow anti-Asian sentiment to boil over, exacerbated by the widely held belief that the virus involved originated in China. In a prime example of "othering," one analysis found that in a two-week period in March 2020, 20% of tweets with the hashtag #covid19 showed anti-Asian sentiments, as did half of those with the hashtag #chinesevirus.[17] "The treatment of Asian Americans is immoral, but also dangerous to public health," wrote Julie Morita in a *Washington Post* essay.[18] An executive vice president at RWJF and the daughter of parents and grandparents sent to internment camps during World War II, Morita called out the damaging health effects of racial hate speech, including its contributions to heart disease, respiratory illness, and other chronic conditions.

Nine months after Morita's essay was published, President Joe Biden condemned the rise in hate crimes and harassment toward Asian Americans during his first public address to the nation.[19] It was not enough to stop them. A brazen shooting attack in several Atlanta spas in mid-March 2021 took eight lives, six of them women of Asian descent. Although the shooter's motives are not fully understood, a potent mix of anti-Asian sentiment and the sexualizing of Asian women appears to have been involved. When Biden traveled to Atlanta to share in the nation's sorrow, the country's first Asian American vice president, Kamala Harris, was by his side. Her very presence, the *New York Times* reported, was "a powerful rejection of the kind of racism and hate" witnessed over the past year, which President Biden said "had to stop. We cannot be complicit. We have to speak out. We have to act."[20]

Those actions, write Mona Shah, PhD, and Tina Kauh, MS, PhD, senior program officers in RWJF's Research-Evaluation-Learning Unit, should include

> increased funding for AAPIs and a new narrative that acknowledges, rather than masks, the vast differences within our community. . . . Conversations across races are essential right now . . . Just as with other Black, Indigenous, and other people of color (BIPOC), Asian Americans suffer from housing and employment discrimination, high rates of uninsurance, and low access to mental health services . . . We stand in solidarity with all communities that have endured racism and discrimination.[21]

Trans Agenda for Liberation

Race and ethnic origin are, of course, only part of the ways in which people identify themselves. Intersectionality theory reminds us that we "contain multitudes," as the poet Walt Whitman would have it, and that we are not defined solely by race, class, gender, or sexuality. Kimberlé Crenshaw, LL.M., JD, Isidor and Seville Sulzbacher Professor of Law at Columbia Law School, who coined the term in the 1990s, describes intersectionality as "a lens through which you can see where power comes and collides, where it interlocks and intersects. It's not simply that there's a race problem here, a gender problem here, and a class or LBGTQ problem there. Many times that framework erases what happens to people who are subject to all of these things."[22]

This is a familiar struggle for the transgender community, said Shelby Chestnut, director of policy and programs at the Transgender Law Center, the country's largest trans-led organization: "Trans people, particularly trans people of color, are just not factored into the conversation. Our work and our narratives and our lived experience are not prioritized."

In 2018, the center convened a group of trans leaders, most of them representing Black, Indigenous, and immigrant communities, to talk about their policy priorities and explore opportunities to gain influence in decision-making settings. "We were expecting them to say, 'we want to be part of these conversations because we often don't have a seat at the table,'" recalled Chestnut. "Instead, what they said really clearly was, 'we don't want to sit at this table anymore. We want to build the table that people come to sit at and we want to set forward the policy priorities. We know the issues impacting our community.'"

From that baseline, the participants crafted the Trans Agenda for Liberation, a five-pillar framework that articulates a campaign for recognition and power.[23] Highlights from that agenda:

- "Black trans women and Black trans femmes living and leading fiercely": In trusting Black trans women to lead, this pillar confronts the violence devastating the community and positions them to drive toward "equitable access to healthcare, housing, bodily autonomy, and intergenerational connection."
- "Beloved home": This elevates the concept that trans people belong, "a movement that honors Native, Indigenous, and Black migrant transgender nonconforming, nonbinary and two spirit peoples . . . where trans people are never forced to leave our homes and we have the freedom of movement to seek out our own belonging."
- "Defining ourselves": This pillar envisions a world in which "our bodies are our own . . . our bodies, HIV statuses, disabilities, and viral loads are no longer policed and criminalized," healthcare is readily available, and self-determination makes it possible to live the fullest lives possible.
- "Intergenerational connection and lifelong care": Recognizing that "our communities are only as strong as our relationships and care for trans people of every age," this pillar describes the building of a movement "that values the beauty of youth and elder wisdom."

- "Freedom to thrive": In demanding safety, rights, and protections for sex workers and "a world without cages," this is a call for "active community support in building lives for ourselves and our families on our own terms."

"We want an agenda that is for and by trans people of color, prioritizing Black leadership and prioritizing people of color," asserted Chestnut, emphasizing the trans community's determination to define its own interests rather than allowing others to define them. But as each contributor to this chapter has emphasized, the intent is not to stand alone: "If we don't work in coalitions broadly across movements, we won't have any wins."

> *None of our issues are separate from one another. If we put them together and fight for each other, we advance trans rights, but also everyone's rights.*
> —Shelby Chestnut

A Final Word

Despite historical injustices, determination may be the characteristic that most fully ties together the many populations that have been pushed to the margins of American society. Yet structural racism continues to create unfairness in our society and economic indicators continue to document the inequitable dispersion of wealth and power. The result is deep harm to Black, Latino, Native American, Asian American, and trans communities. Incomplete data collection too often aggregates broad swaths of the population or omits them altogether, with the result that their stories are not fully told and appropriate policy responses are not advocated for and developed.

In the face of all that, communities are changing the narratives about their own lives and demanding to be heard. Trans people will not be erased, vowed Shelby Chestnut, an assertion that has been widely echoed by others in this chapter as well. They are also insisting, as Nikole Hannah-Jones urged in the previous chapter, that we confront some of our illusions about American history in order to move past them.

That requires naming the problem. The Black Lives Matter movement has made it clear that White supremacy is not only about a small group of extremists but is also reflected in our core institutions. And that, declared Echo Hawk, "is the bigger call to action," the insight that can fuel a larger movement: "If we really understand that there are deep problems in the way that people of color in this country are dehumanized, if we take the opportunity to speak to that, we will all benefit."

A final recollection from Cartagena stands as a source of inspiration in pursuit of that goal. As he tells the story, an older woman who lived through the terrors of World War II remarked: "We are dominant spirits. We are spirits that are meant to survive. All of this stuff is in the way, but there is a beauty about our struggle that is common, regardless of race or wealth. There is the ability to not just survive, but also to thrive."

Keeping It Real

Pathways to Authentic Connections

Beneta D. Burt, MPPA, President and CEO, Mississippi Urban League, Inc.

Gail C. Christopher, D.N., Executive Director, National Collaborative for Health Equity (NCHE); Founder of Ntianu Garden: Center for Healing and Nature; Senior Scholar, Center for the Advancement of Well-Being, George Mason University

Derek M. Griffith, PhD, Co-Founder and Director, Racial Justice Institute; Founder and Director, Center for Men's Health Equity; Professor of Health Systems Administration and Oncology, Georgetown University

Jennifer Gunter, PhD, Director, South Carolina Collaborative on Race, University of South Carolina

Teneasha Washington, PhD, MPH, Assistant Professor, Health Behavior, School of Public Health, University of Alabama at Birmingham

An educator who requested anonymity, an American public school district

An embedded racial hierarchy drives popular narratives about race in the United States and shapes the institutions, systems, and structures that govern our lives (see Chapter 1). While policymakers, the media, and the public have become more familiar with the language and realities of racism in recent years, that foundational hierarchy continues to drive a wedge between people of different races.

Beneta D. Burt, Gail C. Christopher, Derek M. Griffith, Jennifer Gunter, and Teneasha Washington, *Keeping It Real*
In: *Necessary Conversations*. Edited by: Alonzo L. Plough, Oxford University Press. © Robert Wood Johnson Foundation
2022. DOI: 10.1093/oso/9780197641477.003.0004

Sharing authentic stories about their experiences with racism creates an opportunity for mutual understanding, but the process requires much more than casual conversational exchanges. Participants "must be open and willing to entertain a diversity of thought and discover a common ground by going to a *higher* ground," writes Alex Pattakos, PhD, founder of the Global Meaning Institute, an international organization that helps individuals find deeper meaning in their lives and work.[1] "Authentic dialogue cannot and will not happen if we are 'prisoners of our thoughts.'"[2]

The importance of authentic connections that can bring people together was a recurring thread at the *Sharing Knowledge* conference. Multiple presenters spoke about the urgent need to exchange candid ideas about racism in order to guide the country toward racial justice and equity; many are themselves doing the work to make that happen in their own communities. What is missing, they say, are settings in which to listen deeply, connect with others, and search together for solutions.

This chapter largely speaks to the conversations about race and racism that need to occur between Black and White people. Other cross-cultural forums are crucial as well, of course, but here we recognize that "a Black/White binary remains one of the enduring frames through which we consider race in this country," as the previous chapter observed.

In the opening section, contributors examine the importance—and difficulty—of talking honestly about race. Unacknowledged White privilege and White fragility are introduced as the proverbial "elephants in the room," crowding out conversations about inequitable structures and replacing them with visceral expressions of personal feeling.

In a solutions-focused second section, the contributors offer ideas for overcoming barriers. Jennifer Gunter presents the principles underlying the Welcome Table, a signature initiative of the South Carolina Collaborative on Race. Leveraging his research, Derek Griffith, who directs the Racial Justice Initiative at Georgetown University, then describes the conversations about racism that he facilitates to promote shared understanding and improve public health outcomes. Next, Beneta Burt brings a community perspective to her work with the Mississippi Urban League, where she creates safe physical and psychological spaces to support authentic storytelling.

As an academic researcher at the University of Alabama at Birmingham with ties to the community, Teneasha Washington shares her strategies, focusing on improving conversations within academia. Finally, an educational leader describes formal and informal methods to promote authentic conversations on behalf of students in a large, diverse public school district. With certain discussions of race-related topics now banned by public officials, this individual felt forced to contribute anonymously. The chapter concludes with a Spotlight: *Sharing*

Stories to Advance Racial Healing, which presents Gail Christopher's widely used Rx Racial Healing Circles™, designed to foster the human connections necessary to heal the damage inflicted by racism.

Hard Truths

The National Museum of African American History and Culture opened to the public in September 2016—the 19th museum in the Smithsonian Institution family and the only national museum devoted exclusively to documenting African American life, history, and culture. Five years later, the museum, which had pledged to be a space in which to discuss race, equity, and inclusion, had to grapple with one unexpected realization: People did not know how to talk about race.

> *Since the opening of the museum, the number one question people ask us is how to talk about race.*[3]
> —The National Museum of African American History and Culture

This is, perhaps, no surprise: Talking honestly with others about important issues of any kind is rarely easy. Consider how difficult it can be to reconcile differences with family members, discuss religious beliefs, or debate immigration or climate change policies. The fraught and long-standing history of embedded structural racism in the United States makes frank exchanges especially uncomfortable. Understanding why begins by examining the concepts of White privilege and White fragility and the ways in which they obstruct progress.

White Privilege, White Fragility: Unacknowledged but Powerful

The failure of White people to recognize White privilege, and the White fragility that reinforces it, have come into sharp focus in recent scholarship. While there is no consensus definition of these terms, two frameworks help to hone their meaning.

Peggy McIntosh, MA, PhD, a retired Wellesley College scholar, illustrated the concept of White privilege by listing the assumptions she can make as a White person that are closed to someone who is Black: "I can if I wish arrange to be in the company of people of my race most of the time." "I can be sure that if I need legal or medical help, my race will not work against me." "I can choose blemish cover or bandages in 'flesh' color and have them more or less match my skin."[4]

*I have come to see White privilege as an invisible package of unearned as-
sets that I can count on cashing in each day, but about which I was "meant"
to remain oblivious. White privilege is like an invisible weightless knapsack
of special provisions, maps, passports, codebooks, visas, clothes, tools, and
blank checks.*

—Peggy McIntosh

White fragility is essentially the response when that privilege is questioned
or challenged. "These moves include the outward display of emotions such as
anger, fear, and guilt, and behaviors such as argumentation, silence, and leaving
the stress-inducing situation. These behaviors, in turn, function to reinstate
White racial equilibrium."[5]

Ignorance about the special place that Whites have been given in American
society does not necessarily mean that someone is indifferent to prejudice.
Quite the contrary, in many cases. While some White people are explicitly racist,
others wear their support of civil rights as a badge of pride. The worldview of
both groups, however, too often remains narrowly tethered to considerations of
individual circumstances, rather than to the structural forces that shaped those
circumstances. "Just as systemic racism is reduced to individual bad actors, privilege is misunderstood as something individual rather than a system in which
White people as a collective are centered and prioritized," reads an October
2020 posting from the University of Central Florida.[6]

Black people, who experience racism at both a personal and a structural level,
tend to seek broad solutions to overhaul systems that privilege Whites. The
White response to the topic of race, by contrast, is often much more personal,
expressed with statements like "I have lots of Black friends" and "I was raised not
to discriminate." Uncomfortable with the suggestion that they are participating
in a system that is stacked against Black people, they default to emotion rather
than having to confront racist structures that enable their advantages. "You have
to acknowledge that you benefit from a system that other people don't benefit
from," said Teneasha Washington, referencing White privilege. "That is very
hard for people to come to terms with."

In general, White people think of racist actions as active efforts to discriminate by, say, keeping Black people out of certain neighborhoods or preventing
them from getting a job, explained Jennifer Gunter, pointing out that passive
racism can be just as damaging but is harder to see. "Some people are so used to
privilege that equality feels like oppression,"[7] observed Lorenzo M. Boyd, PhD,
assistant provost of diversity and inclusion at the University of New Haven in
Connecticut.

Until there is a national reckoning with the systemic harms caused by
racism, conversations about the topic will remain clouded in tensions and

misunderstandings. The result is frustrating to participants of both races—a strain that contributors variously describe as mired in fear, shame, guilt, avoidance, and denial.

Common Tensions: Fear, Shame, Guilt, Avoidance, Denial

The challenge to authentic conversations is grounded in the struggle to find the right words and then not being afraid to use them. "Because our area is so diverse, people of color and Whites are fearful to engage in that conversation for fear of political missteps," said the educator who asked not to be identified Beneta Burt notices the same fear when facilitating conversations in her community: "It's very hard to have an honest conversation. Some White people will think you believe they are being racist. Some Black people will think you believe they are being radical."

White people who perceive equity as a zero–sum game—*if someone else gets ahead, I lose ground*—may be afraid of losing gains they have secured or of being accused of not deserving what they feel they have earned. "You feel like you are losing something . . . you are losing your privilege to something," Teneasha Washington said, characterizing White fragility.

A familiar claim made by White people is that they are "colorblind." Burt reports hearing people say, "I think everybody is equal. I just don't see race." Another common refrain—"I didn't cause this situation and I am certainly not a racist"—allows Whites to deny their complicity in racial injustice and turn away from any obligation to participate in dismantling systems of racial oppression.

These non-starters to true conversations can be difficult to confront. People of color are sometimes reluctant to introduce issues they think will suggest to Whites that they are overly sensitive or "touchy." They may also hold back on using the blunt language of White privilege and fragility, fearing that it will make White people stop listening and turn away from dialogue.

Instead, Black people sometimes "lead from behind," with the goal of getting all voices heard. "People of color have to be willing to not say anything, because when we talk too much, other people don't want to say anything," observed Washington. In her work with community members, Burt has come to recognize how important it is for Black people to hear other perspectives. While it is hard to hear inaccurate views, she has found that the best path forward is sometimes "being able to sit, listen, and be willing to hear the hard issues from others."

The ability to have a genuine conversation is further complicated by shame. "So many people carry some sense of shame and guilt when it comes to race and racism," said Gunter. "Whether our forefathers caused the harm or received the harm, we carry this shame, and when we experience the shame, we shut down."

Even those who aspire to forge deep connections that allow Black people and White people to reach a place of shared understanding find authentic dialogue to be a struggle. Shifting to more neutral terms, such as social justice or social determinants of health (often without acknowledging that racism is one of those determinants), is one way that people avoid directly confronting the issues. "Often, if you bring up racism, the conversation shifts to social determinants and things that are more comfortable to discuss," said Derek Griffith.

Likewise, there is a tendency to blur "equity," which recognizes that adjustments of some kind are needed, given racial differences in access to opportunities and pervasive obstacles to being healthy, and "equality," which dictates that everyone should be given the same access to opportunity, regardless of their starting place. Thus, "equality lenses 'psychologize' racial inequities and suggest that racial differences in health outcomes are because of racial differences in effort, motivation, tenacity, and other intrapersonal characteristics," added Griffith. Elevating the equity framework can be unfamiliar or threatening to many White people, yet it is the true path forward.

Why Talking Is So Important

No matter how disquieting, the need for authentic conversation is vital. When they work, exchanges about difficult issues can yield enormous personal growth and create a path to positive community and societal transformation.

Uncomfortable experiences often lead to change, agreed Brian Lowery, PhD, senior associate dean at Stanford University's Graduate School of Business, who studies the psychology of racial privilege. "When people are willing to accept that privilege exists . . . when you give them the opportunity to talk . . . there's reason to believe that they might actually support policies that dismantle it or work against it," he said.[8]

In an insight as profound as it is crisp, the contributors argue that it is important to have these deep discussions because we know what the country looks like when they don't happen—we are witnessing the fractures that result. "Not having these conversations has gotten us to where we are right now," said Jennifer Gunter. And, as multiple chapters in this book illustrate, "where we are right now" is in a country mired in inequity and violence, driven by resentment and rage. Long-standing racial, social, and economic problems remain unresolved, distrust of leaders and institutions runs deep, and divisions mask our many commonalities. In the absence of broad commitments to pursue genuine structural change, activists have taken to the streets to protest police violence toward people of color and elevated the urgency of the Black Lives Matter movement. Declaring that the racial discrimination embedded in American society and its deadly consequences for Black people is unacceptable, they have brought home a singular exigency: We must figure out how to talk to one another about race and racism. In this next section, the contributors discuss how they are working to make these critical conversations happen.

Changing the Narrative in South Carolina

Jennifer Gunter, a native Mississippian, believes in the power of stories to illuminate the present, facilitate healing, and forge a better future. Gunter's early work as an historian grew out of her mother's advocacy on behalf of women's rights. "The women's movement happened in every town in every state," she recalled. "Women met with each other, they had conversations," and with them came the insights and growth needed to transform norms.

> We believe that open and honest conversations have the ability to heal communities.
>
> —Jennifer Gunter

Gunter's philosophy and the conversations she facilitates propose a "call-in" culture that asks people to talk about how they developed their perspectives. A call-in culture, as outlined by Loretta J. Ross,[9] allows for conversations that help people see and indict underlying structural inequities. A "call-out" culture, by contrast, reduces the issue to an individual problem.

Today, Gunter directs the South Carolina Collaborative on Race at the University of South Carolina. Established in 2015 after the mass killings at Mother Emanuel AME Church in Charleston, the collaborative puts inclusivity at the center of its mission as it works to "foster racial reconciliation and civic renewal through ongoing dialogues in classrooms, boardrooms, and community rooms."[10]

The collaborative's principles of education, facilitation, and connection weave through all of its projects, which engage youth, law enforcement, educators, community organizers, and many others. A key goal is to bring the widest possible range of voices to any activity—Black people and White people, people who have disabilities, and others from a diverse range of ethnic and socioeconomic backgrounds. "When we work with communities, we really work with them to think about whose voice might be missing, who else is part of this community," Gunter believes.

The Welcome Table

One of the collaborative's core projects is the Welcome Table, which uses stories to build trust among people and communities interested in addressing racial and ethnic divisions and working for positive change. The Welcome Table builds on an innovative framework "designed to transform biased mindsets and inequitable systems," and owes its development to Susan Glisson, PhD, founding executive director of the William Winter Institute for Racial Reconciliation. Glisson, in turn, credits the work to those who have come before, leaving us their lessons and wisdom, such as Chuck McDew, Ella Baker, and Fannie Lou Hamer.

The Welcome Table features "a series of carefully scaffolded activities that are based in storytelling . . . sharing who your authentic self is, reconnecting with your core values so you can see them reflected back to you," explained Gunter. Sometimes, the process includes small-group discussions about a suggested topic that allow people to talk intimately—for example, exploring the framework of structural racism and the myth of colorblind ideology. Another strategy is to give each person a specified length of time to talk without interruption, "to demonstrate that all voices are equally valuable."

Authentic conversations can lead to moving "ah-ha" moments, Gunter has learned. In one, a Blackman described "the specific way" he had to attend to his hair and dress before leaving home so that he was not immediately profiled because of his race. The response from the White people in the room was a sense of disbelief and confusion that this had often occurred. "They were like, 'there's no way that happened to you.' And he was like, 'you know, it does happen to me,'" said Gunter. That moment, and others like it, open people's minds, she said.

> *People around the state are finally having conversations with one another about how race impacts their work. When we give permission to talk about race, it opens up a floodgate.*
>
> —Jennifer Gunter

Conversations to Advance Public Health Goals

Like Gunter, Derek Griffith hails from the South and leverages his position in academia to promote racial justice. His commitment is rooted in the childhood experience of being one among only a handful of Black children attending a private school in the Atlanta area. Recalling that experience as the moment he became fascinated with the idea of racism, Griffith said, "It didn't make a lot of sense to me that you make a judgment about a whole group of people you don't really know about and have never really met."

This fascination led him first to study the emergence of Black social activists and then to his current position as director of the newly formed Racial Justice Institute at Georgetown University in Washington, D.C. Griffith's research focuses especially on developing interventions to mitigate the effects of racism and the risk of chronic disease among Black men. He also develops and tests anti-racism interventions in public health departments.

Through trainings and facilitated discussions, Griffith helps to guide public health officials and practitioners to make the connection between racism and health outcomes and apply that understanding to their professional roles and responsibilities. Not everyone in public health or other disciplines may be equally invested in a broad vision of racial justice, Griffith acknowledges, but most health professionals embrace insights that will help them do their own work more effectively.

Dealing with the terminology of race and racism is an essential first step, he believes. "We have to understand that racism implies that differences in health are due to intrinsic racial differences, not different access to opportunities and resources and different amounts of exposure to stress," he said, joining other contributors in emphasizing the connections between individual experiences and the structural racism that enables White privilege.

> *Structural racism is a process of looking at how patterns that may not seem connected are actually shaping things that happen over time.*
>
> —Derek Griffith

Griffith's experience facilitating discussions has taught him the perils of erecting walls versus the value of building bridges. "People are not going to agree with things because they are factually correct; they will dismiss it as inaccurate information," he observed. Taking our focus away from characterizing patterns and structures as racism to labeling people as racist often is distracting and for many just creates "a wall that is difficult for them to get over."

Promoting shared understanding and empathy instead allows people to "feel" someone else's experiences more deeply and to look beyond themselves and tame the White fragility that closes minds. "Hitting people in the heart" is important to building sustainable bridges, Griffith said, an observation that grounds much of Gail C. Christopher's work as well (see the Spotlight at the end of this chapter).

The Power of Stories on the Ground

As president and CEO of the Mississippi Urban League, Mississippi-born Beneta Burt is as familiar as Griffith with the challenges in local communities. Formed in 2018 through a merger with the nonprofit Mississippi Roadmap to Health Equity, which Burt directed since its inception in 2003, the Mississippi Urban League is a one-stop community-based organization for people seeking help with employment, education, housing, health, and other services.

Although conversations about race are more common today than when she was a child, Burt recognizes that people still have trouble accepting the existence of racism and do not take readily to the notion that some people "started out way ahead."

In a repurposed former grocery store in Jackson, Burt helped to create a safe space where Black people can meet and talk among themselves and with White people about rooting out structural racism. The facility, developed after a series of community-based conversations about local priorities, also features a state-of-the-art fitness center, a food pantry, and a kitchen.

In that comfortable gathering space, Burt facilitates dialogue in a calm manner that "allows people room to be uncomfortable and allows them room to respond and ask questions of you, questions which might make you uncomfortable as well. You just have to keep talking."

> *Having a conversation about race is not about blaming all White people for slavery and its consequences, but rather about acknowledging the existence of slavery and its consequences.*
>
> —Beneta Burt

Her goal in guiding people past their unease is to encourage Whites to begin asking what they can do to topple structures and institutions that harm Black people. Fostering comfort allows those kinds of authentic conversations to take place, she believes: "People have to have some degree of comfort about who is at the table" in order to enter conversations with open minds.

As these gatherings move closer to understanding what racial reconciliation requires, Burt sometimes offers a gentle rejoinder to that familiar claim of some White people: "I don't see color."

"I wake up Black every day," Burt says. "You just wake up."

That reminder demonstrates an engagement with community members that goes far deeper than what typically occurs when White people reach out to Black people because a funder or research design has called in vague terms for "community input." On those occasions, Burt says, there may be "polite applause after a presentation," but the more honest conversation—"the real meeting"—happens after the White people leave.

Like Gunter, Burt believes in the power of stories to illustrate the pain of being Black in the United States and offers her own experience as a vehicle for positive change. Heeding advice from friends and colleagues to "put on your armor," she talks about the ways in which she feels compelled to be "on" all the time, to be more prepared for meetings than anyone else, and to take extraordinary precautions to avoid even a small misstep, knowing that her ideas or perspectives are likely to be overlooked or dismissed. Burt tries to share those experiences with others, urging that they respond "in a way to reach for the heartstrings" so that people "understand that race really matters, and racism is there."

Pursuing Equity in Academic Settings

Teneasha Washington, a public health professor and researcher at the University of Alabama at Birmingham, challenges the notion that conversations about racism are inevitably touchy. "We should be able to have a meaningful conversation . . . it's not really a conversation of sensitivity," she insists. Rather, it is a conversation that asks: "How do we progressively change the momentum around racism? Because we know it clearly exists."

Washington believes academic institutions have a responsibility to foster dialogue about racism as a component of their service mission yet struggle to do so, in part because their own track record is far from stellar. Most academic settings deliver more professional benefit to those who conduct research and publications than to those who serve on academic committees or promote authentic conversations about racism within the university, Washington believes. Yet responsibility for guiding those efforts tends to fall disproportionately—and unfairly—on Black faculty and other faculty of color. "We should be able to allow other people to step into that space and address that issue because oftentimes, they live in the world that benefits," she argued. "It is everybody's job to be able to facilitate those conversations."

> *The dominant culture has to take a very big role in dismantling racism. It doesn't always have to fall on a minority.*
>
> —Teneasha Washington

The perception of faculty as elite individuals to be held in high esteem makes it especially challenging to be honest about enduring racism. But privilege needs to be acknowledged, even though it means White people may be asked to concede that their achievements reflect more than just their talent. "It's kind of breaking down that you may not be where you are just because of who you are in your field," Washington said.

Non-Whites who are successful in academia face other kinds of constraints, with their success putting them in a double bind: They may not be comfortable expressing concerns about racism because their achievements signal they have overcome barriers, yet they are expected to lead and educate others on the issues.

A hard look at all of that needs to be part of candid, two-way conversations, said Washington: "For me to be authentic, I also have to allow other people to be authentic." Being able to reach a place where people can openly disagree is not a sign of failure, as long as it is respectful disagreement, she noted. Rather, it is an indication that some level of authenticity has been achieved.

Asking a White person to speak first can be a strategy to ease into difficult conversations, Washington suggested, because White people sometimes disengage if they feel under attack as Black people talk about persistent racism. Ultimately, everyone needs permission to share their experiences frankly and to recognize that one person cannot invalidate the perceptions of another. "Every voice must be heard even if that creates tension or dissension," she urged. "I can just say how I feel in my space."

Another issue that carries particular weight in academia is how research studies or other activities that involve community members are conducted. A strong advocate for the communities of Birmingham, where she earned her degrees, Washington often facilitates conversations aimed at removing power imbalances and leveling the playing field between the university and local residents. One strategy to build relationships is relinquishing power and demonstrating humility. "I leave my titles and degrees at the door," she said, so that other voices can be elevated. Recognizing that the often-overlooked contributions of community residents are also important, she makes it a point to include their bylines in reports and dissemination efforts.

Candor in a Public School District

Starting conversations about race and equity has been a touchstone of one educational leader's career. That work, focused on equity and diversity in a public school district that serves multiple cities, promotes candid exchanges in an environment of mutual respect. "When you try to understand *their* perspectives, people are more willing to understand *your* perspective," said the educator. Nonetheless, as noted, this individual asked not to be identified because public policies in the region are increasingly constraining the dialogue.

To bring attention to inequities in the school district, they knew it was important to combine students' stories with solid local data on the disproportionate rates of suspensions, expulsions, and arrests among students of color. Data helped stakeholders see the effects of structural racism on student achievement. "We can't inspire people to exceed expectations if we reinforce negative concepts about who they are and what they're capable of," this individual said. Making data public has also been key to initiating change in the district, as has the school board's willingness "to publicly put out data that doesn't always paint a pretty picture."

Following a public tragedy, the educator saw that the district's Black and Brown students needed to talk about how responses to violence differ depending on who the victims are, but also realized that many teachers did not feel equipped to guide that kind of race-based conversation. The missing resource was provided by Courageous Conversations™[11], a course developed by the Pacific Educational Group that guides systems and organizations "to address racial disparities through safe, authentic, and effective cross-racial dialogue."

Facilitated by a person in each school, the course became a resource for teachers and a tool for guiding discussion. Participants learn how to use "four key agreements" and "six essential conditions" to talk about race through a framework designed "to help individuals and organizations address persistent racial disparities intentionally, explicitly, and comprehensively." Said the educator, "I think that has been helpful in creating a synergy around people's willingness to work with kids in these conversations. It allowed us to move forward."

> *Those who are benefiting from the marginalization of others have to be the ones to recognize it and publicly speak to it when it happens.*
>
> —Local educator

A Final Word

This much is clear: Authentic conversations about racism are difficult, uncomfortable, and happening far too infrequently. But as this chapter and its contributors show, the question "How do we talk about racism?" is finally being asked. In boardrooms and cultural spaces, at home and among friends, in houses of workshop and educational settings, there are signs that people want to talk authentically about racism and are eager for guidance.

Through authentic connections, people have an opportunity to reconsider and challenge the zero–sum thinking that has buttressed structural racism and hindered equity. In her 2021 book *The Sum of Us*, Heather McGhee illustrates the ways White people undermine their own well-being when they fail to join in cross-racial solidarity to advance equitable strategies that benefit everyone. Traveling throughout the United States, McGhee uses real-life stories, economic data, and historical incidents to make this case, highlighting the urgency and value of talking authentically across racial lines to tackle a multitude of social justice issues.

A 2020 Monmouth University poll revealed that 76% of Americans and 71% of White Americans believe that racial and ethnic discrimination is a "big problem" in this country.[12] The same year, the National Museum of African American History and Culture launched "Talking About Race," an online portal to help individuals, families, and communities explore racism, racial identity, and the ways these forces shape every aspect of society.

Clearly, many Americans now recognize the imperative to tackle racism with an open heart and a curious mind. And as contributors throughout this book also indicate, perhaps—just perhaps—individuals and policymakers are beginning to act as well.

Spotlight

Sharing Stories to Advance Racial Healing

Gail C. Christopher, D.N., Executive Director, National Collaborative for Health Equity (NCHE), Founder of Ntianu Garden: Center for Healing and Nature, Senior Scholar, George Mason University, Center for the Advancement of Well-Being

Everyone has biases—some are innate while others are learned. Yet, not everyone acts harmfully toward others as a result of those biases. What makes the difference, one program suggests, is human connection.

Gail C. Christopher designed Rx Racial Healing Circles™ to foster those human connections. Using the ancient practice of circles and the modern science of emotional intelligence, the program brings together diverse groups through facilitated storytelling to share personal truths and build empathy among participants.

> *To be biased is not to be racist. To be biased is to be human because the brain has to categorize things based on the stories that it receives.*
>
> —Gail C. Christopher

Rx Racial Healing Circles™ are framed around the belief that every person in America has been hurt by the false ideology of a racial hierarchy and so everyone has work to do to heal. That work can be difficult, because it is often hard to share stories about race without shutting down or psychologically disengaging, but the rewards can be profound.

For the last four decades, Christopher has been building social programs that promote racial healing and relationship building, which is the centerpiece of the Truth, Racial Healing and Transformation (TRHT) framework. Launched by W.K. Kellogg Foundation with other philanthropic organizations in 2016,

Gail C. Christopher, *Spotlight* In: *Necessary Conversations*. Edited by: Alonzo L. Plough, Oxford University Press. © Robert Wood Johnson Foundation 2022. DOI: 10.1093/oso/9780197641477.003.0005

TRHT is a national movement that urges the nation to embrace its "common humanity" and eliminate racial inequities.

To further the impact of her work, Christopher helped to form the Rx Racial Healing Circles™ Collaborative in 2018.[1] A year later, she became executive director at the National Collaborative for Health Equity, where she uses a national platform to share the healing circles.

When Christopher describes the Rx Racial Healing Circles™ at conferences and institutions across the nation, she invariably captures audiences with her small stature, big smile, and bold message. Her optimism is contagious and her hope for an America that follows its foundational truth that all are created equal is inspirational. In her own graceful storytelling style, Christopher describes a tragic personal experience—the loss of a child in a biased healthcare system. At the same time, she acknowledges her own biases, describing behavior toward a home remodeling contractor that embarrassed her deeply.

With that narrative, she models the power of truthful stories to build empathy and create a pathway to healing and transformation. In her wrap-up, she issues a call for everyone to work toward racial healing for the sake of children of color— the majority of young people in his country.

Framework for Expanding Empathy and Building Relationships

Rx Racial Healing Circles™ bring together small groups from public, private, and nonprofit organizations with trained facilitators. Using a methodology that stresses active learning and being open to the perspectives and experiences of others, the circles are designed to be as diverse as possible, across race, age, gender, and geographic lines. Following an introductory exercise, participants pair off for deep discussion around a strategic prompt and then share their stories with the whole group.

An ancient practice used by Indigenous peoples during storytelling gatherings, circles are known for their healing properties.[2] Christopher says these circles promote three assets—appreciation, belonging, and consciousness change.

Appreciation is associated with feeling thankful and being affirmed. Trust builds as participants share narratives, learn to listen to one another, and become confident that they are being heard. Science supports the benefits—researchers at the HeartMath Institute, which develops scientifically based tools to bridge the connection between heart and mind, has published research indicating that feeling appreciated leads to a state of harmony.[3]

Creating the sense of belonging that is a basic human need is another power of circles. They provide an opportunity for participants to be equal and to not only see one another, but also to see themselves in the other through stories, Christopher explained.

Finally, consciousness change is a key aim for facilitators who are tasked with using emotional intelligence to guide participants in exercises aimed at "de-biasing." Heart and mind are both engaged in the work of replacing false narratives about "perceived others" with true stories about one human race. As participants connect with the stories of others, their brains form a new schema that diminishes thoughts that drive separation or difference and replaces them with thoughts of empathy and connectedness.

Through appreciation, belonging, and consciousness change, Christopher says, groups can practice empathy to "peel back layers of denial and come face to face with our true humanity."

> We can stand up as American people and learn to see ourselves in the face of each other. We can learn to demonstrate empathy and compassion for one another.
>
> —Gail C. Christopher

The circles are not a substitute for other approaches to racial healing, she emphasizes. Rather, they complement other efforts to achieve racial justice and increase needed levels of public will and engagement. "Protests, policy, and practice changes, as well as accountability, are also required," explained Christopher.

The success of Rx Racial Healing Circles™ is evident in the footprints they are leaving across the nation. Christopher has trained hundreds of professionals to co-facilitate the approach in more than a dozen institutions. Committed to ensuring lasting impact, she continues to offer trainings virtually and in-person and recently wrote Rx Racial Healing: A Guide to Our Humanity, published by the Association of American Colleges & Universities, to train others in implementing racial healing circles that use her methodology. As well, her work has inspired U.S. lawmakers to propose important resolutions calling for the creation of a Commission on Truth, Racial Healing, and Transformation,[4] which is inspired by truth commissions implemented by over 40 nations to confront conflicts resulting from government injustice.

PART II

THE HARMS OF RACIAL INJUSTICE

To explore the influence of racial injustice on health, this section drills down to specific population groups, examining the health inequities imposed on Black women, incarcerated people, and immigrants in the first three chapters. It concludes with a chapter that exposes the disproportionate impact of the climate crisis on people of color, described by one contributor as "the hard truths of what racism has done." The deep-seated disparities that accompanied the COVID-19 pandemic are considered throughout, underscoring the health and economic burdens that have been shouldered by the most vulnerable populations.

With race already situated as an important social determinant of health earlier in this book, Chapter 4, "Structural Racism in Black Maternal Healthcare," grapples with the historical harm inflicted on Black women by the very systems that should contribute to their health and well-being. The structural racism embedded in the healthcare system has produced a Black infant mortality rate that is double that of White infants and a significantly higher death rate from pregnancy-related causes among Black women. As it translates statistics into personal stories and experiences, this chapter documents the continuing harms stemming from a legacy of medical racism.

Chapter 5, "The Health Harms of Incarceration and Punishment," weaves together examples of carceral injustice and structural racism in a country that incarcerates more people—and a higher percentage of its population—than any other nation in the world. Groundbreaking research conducted on Medicaid health data on New York City's Rikers

Island jail complex and first-person accounts of deplorable conditions inside Mississippi state prisons highlight the consequences of incarceration and punishment for individuals and their families and communities. Those realities drove RWJF's decision in 2018 to measure incarceration as a social determinant of health and well-being.

Racism and discrimination dominate the lives of so many immigrants in this country as well. Chapter 6, "Immigrant Health: Inequity and Fear," draws on stories of immigrants and undocumented individuals, from the Mexican-U.S. border to rural communities in Illinois, to give a human face to the effects of cruel rhetoric and punitive public policies. Data that show rising rates of cancer, heart disease, and depression in communities faced with deportation threats and constant Immigration and Customs Enforcement (ICE) raids highlight the urgent need for a more humane approach.

Chapter 7, "Climate Crisis, Environmental Justice, and Racial Justice," concludes this section by positioning the climate crisis as a primary source of racial inequity and explores the sustained efforts of the environmental justice movement to change that. Contributors describe the front-line challenges facing a resilient Alaskan community; explain the connections among water equity, health equity, and climate injustice; and explore the intersection of the climate crisis and COVID-19. A leading next-generation voice talks about the role that youth are playing in the climate justice movement, bringing the chapter to a close on a note of hope.

4

Structural Racism in Black Maternal Healthcare

Shana Bartley, MSPH, Director of Community Partnerships, Income Security and Child Care/Early Learning, National Women's Law Center

Susan Beane, MD, Executive Medical Director, Healthfirst

Nakeitra Burse, DrPH, CHES, CEO, Six Dimensions, LLC

Joia Crear-Perry, MD, FACOG, Founder & President, National Birth Equity Collaborative

Linda Villarosa, MA, Assistant Professor of Media Communication & Arts and Black Studies at the City College of New York and contributing writer to the New York Times Magazine

In 1619, the first Africans were brought to the United States on slave ships, launching the brutal institution of slavery in this country, an institution marked by the inhumane assault on the bodies and minds of Black women, men, and children. The weight of centuries of such treatment, both supported by and embedded into the structure of medical care and the healthcare system itself, can be felt more than 400 years later in the health status of Black people and in their experiences with healthcare providers and the healthcare system today. Experiences that should advance their health and well-being instead too often exacerbate long-standing injustices.

Historical maltreatment, structural racism, and the physical and psychological demands of "living while Black" have had a damaging impact on the health of childbearing women and their infants. From prenatal care to labor and delivery, from the postpartum period to child care, the healthcare system's underlying

Shana Bartley, Susan Beane, Nakeitra Burse, Joia Crear-Perry, and Linda Villarosa, *Structural Racism in Black Maternal Healthcare* In: *Necessary Conversations*. Edited by: Alonzo L. Plough, Oxford University Press. © Robert Wood Johnson Foundation 2022. DOI: 10.1093/oso/9780197641477.003.0006

racial biases have denied Black women the resources and attention they need and deserve.

The contributors to this chapter, who are themselves Black women, bring historical knowledge, contextual perspective, and personal experience as they address the harms of structural racism in maternal healthcare. Journalist Linda Villarosa offers a context rooted in history for considering Black women's health and their interactions with the U.S. healthcare system today. Obstetrician/gynecologist and advocate Joia Crear-Perry of the National Birth Equity Collaborative (NBEC) deepens our understanding of the role of bias and structural racism on Black maternal healthcare, while public health practitioner Nakeitra Burse explores the personal impact of racial bias on the birth experiences of Black women. Susan Beane, Healthfirst executive medical director, describes interventions in the city and state of New York while Shana Bartley from the National Women's Law Center extends the discussion to the experience of child-care users and workers. Finally, in a spotlight, Beane describes a partnership between a health plan and a health system to help marginalized women achieve better postnatal health outcomes.

Centuries of Harm by People and Systems

Four hundred years after those first Africans reached the shore of Virginia, the racism that has permeated the treatment of Black women's bodies continues to impact their health and experiences of pregnancy, childbirth, and the post-partum period.

The evidence is clear in stark mortality data:

- **Black infants are significantly more likely to die than White infants.** The Black infant mortality rate is 2.3 times that of White infants.[1]
- **Black women are significantly more likely to die from pregnancy-related causes than White women.** From 2014 to 2017 non-Hispanic Black women in the United States died from pregnancy-related causes at a rate of 41.7 per 100,000 live births, a rate 3.1 times that of non-Hispanic White women (13.4 per 100,000).[2] Causes of death most often include cardiac conditions, preeclampsia and eclampsia, hemorrhage, and embolism.[3]
- **Education, income, and access to healthcare do not protect Black birthing people from the risk of maternal death.** The publicly discussed birth experiences of tennis icon Serena Williams[4] and superstar Beyoncé,[5] and those of many other educated Black women with good health insurance and access to quality healthcare, underscore this fact. Black women with

college degrees have a higher risk of experiencing a preterm birth than White women who did not graduate from high school.[6]

- **The maternal health outcomes of Black women play out against a broader set of grim Black health outcomes data.** Black people in the United States are 60% more likely to be diagnosed with diabetes,[7] 50% more likely to have a stroke,[8] 40% more likely to have high blood pressure, and 20% more likely to die from heart disease[9] than non-Hispanic White people. Black people also have the highest death rates for all cancers combined and for most major cancers of any racial and ethnic group.[10]

Is there something about the Black body that causes this increased risk of infant and maternal mortality? Or does it primarily reflect the social conditions of their lives and the disregard of institutions charged with their care? With the first question asked and answered—biology is not a factor—the second must be explored to understand health inequities more fully.

> *If Black people's education and their wealth don't protect them, it must be something else. We rely on clinical answers while either ignoring, downplaying, or giving lip service to the lived experience of being a Black woman in America.*
>
> —Linda Villarosa

Racist American institutions, systems, and structures enabled horrific physical treatment of Black women to meet the financial interests of slave owners seeking more enslaved labor, physicians experimenting with new surgical techniques and justification for flawed medical ideas, and social engineers hoping to reduce the Black population.

For 250 years, on slave auction blocks throughout the South—and in the North as well until 1804—young Black women were prodded in front of bustling crowds so that prospective buyers could test their health, strength, and potential for producing healthy babies for more enslaved labor.[11]

J. Marion Sims performed gynecological surgery without anesthesia on three enslaved women–Anarcha, Betsy, and Lucy. Subscribing to the myth that Black people could better tolerate pain, he forced his studies on non-consenting adults in the hopes of developing new surgical techniques.[12] Sims has been vilified for these procedures yet also lauded as the "father of gynecology."[13] The *New York Times* noted, "One would be hard pressed to find a more controversial figure in the history of medicine than J. Marion Sims."[14]

In an example of the rampant racism within the medical system in 1960s Mississippi, Fannie Lou Hamer, a key voice in the civil rights movement, received a nonconsensual hysterectomy in 1961 by a White doctor while under-going surgery for a uterine tumor. So common was the forced sterilization of Black women, intended to reduce the Black population, that it earned the moniker "a Mississippi appendectomy."[15] According to Hamer's own research, "about six out of the 10 Negro women that go to the [county] hospital are sterilized with the tubes tied."[16]

The legacy of this medical racism endures, surfacing today in the health status of Black people, in their treatment by clinicians, and in their own fears and attitudes toward the healthcare system. Today, some Black people are reluctant to receive the COVID-19 vaccine as an understandable response to centuries of negative experiences with medical providers and the healthcare system.

Through her public health consulting company Six Dimensions, Nakeitra Burse has produced a documentary film, *Laboring with Hope*, that translates statistics into stories.[17] The film draws on Burse's own family—her aunt died after giving birth, her sister-in-law died three weeks after childbirth, and her sister has had two miscarriages and lost an eight-month-old baby, which is considered a case of infant mortality—to remind viewers that the effects of racism are experienced at the most personal levels. Burse screens the film with the goal of spurring action on maternal health.

Understanding race as a social construct, not a biological fact, is key to appreciating that none of this is preordained. (See Chapter 1, which presents a taxonomy of race constructed in the 1700s that endured into the 20th century.) "We need to be able to see that we're all one human race," stressed Joia Crear-Perry, founder and president of NBEC. "There is no Black gene, no Asian gene. Racism has made these hierarchies and castes and boxes that don't fit who we really are."

> There's nothing innately broken about different groups of people based on their skin color. But when they are treated differently, when they're valued differently, their health outcomes will reflect that.
>
> —Joia Crear-Perry

Myths That Endure and Continue to Injure

The assumptions of the past continue to influence contemporary medical treatment. For example, the misconception that Black people have a higher pain tolerance than Whites has not been fully set aside by many healthcare workers. A 2019 study of women undergoing cesarean sections (C-sections) found that Black women were assessed less frequently for pain and given lower doses of pain medication than White women, despite higher pain scores following surgery.[18]

The reflexive resistance to giving Black patients less pain medication than White patients[19] dovetails neatly with stereotypes of Black people who request pain medication as drug seekers or sellers.[20]

Another myth that puts women at risk is that blood pressure "runs high" in Black people, which can affect timely assessment and treatment of high blood pressure during pregnancy and childbirth and afterwards. The results are potentially dire, as high blood pressure can be a sign of preeclampsia and eclampsia, potentially lethal pregnancy and postpartum conditions. "The biases in our head end up being deadly for our patients," said Crear-Perry.

Whether intentional or structural, the racism underlying these kinds of medical responses has put the lives of Black childbearing women and their infants at risk.

"Weathering" and Black Women's Childbirth Experience

Arline T. Geronimus, ScD, professor at the University of Michigan School of Public Health, has coined the term "weathering," essentially an accelerated aging process, to describe the impact of life experiences on a Black woman's body.[21] Geronimus observed that the infants of Black teen mothers were more likely to survive than infants of Black mothers in their 20s and 30s, which are considered optimal childbearing years. By contrast, the infants of White teen mothers fare worse than those of older White mothers. Geronimus proposed the "weathering hypothesis" to explain this difference, positing that Black women's health may decline in early adulthood "as a physical consequence of cumulative socioeconomic disadvantage."

Speaking to the "weathering in Black women and the social pressure of being a Black woman," Burse observed, "There's no room to get tired or process your feelings. We are always ensuring that those we love and care about are taken care of." Acknowledging the "strong Black woman" stereotype, Burse added, "I want our strength to be applauded, but I don't want the world to depend on it."

The impact of racism on maternal health and the experiences of pregnant and postpartum Black women can undermine the joy of pregnancy. "Pregnancy is almost this supernatural experience," said Burse. "You're growing a human being and there's excitement and that happy feeling that most women get, whether it's planned or unplanned." But for Black women the challenges of interacting with the healthcare system and finding providers who will listen to them loom large. Black women must "arm ourselves with information and strategies to try to make it home," Burse stressed. It is an emotionally and physically complex task, she admitted, "to figure out how to take care of myself in a system that I fear won't take care of me."

The biggest issue is Black women not being listened to in the healthcare system.

—Nakeitra Burse

One manifestation of the system's failure to meet the needs of Black women is the reluctance among Black women to breastfeed. Arguably, that can be traced, at least in part, to the era when enslaved women were required to use their breast milk to nourish their master's children, rather than their own.[22] The resentment and disconnect engendered by that experience has lasted over the centuries, exacerbated by other structural faults in present times. Too often, Burse observed, Black women are just given formula to feed their babies in the hospital, with no discussion of breastfeeding and its value.

The broad challenge of creating better pregnancy, childbirth, and postpartum experiences for Black women reflects a fundamental lack of attention to root causes and the failure to address the issue with the urgency it demands. "We have data, we have stories—and yet Black women are still not a priority," stated Burse with frustration.

The bias that invades all parts of our society also shows up in the experiences of Blacks and other people of color when we enter the healthcare system.

—Linda Villarosa

On the Path to Maternal Health Equity

There are many inflection points where it becomes possible to shift from a healthcare system characterized by bias, exclusion, inattention, and (at worst) cruelty toward Black women to one committed to recognizing and supporting their autonomy and individual needs before, during, and after childbirth. People from many sectors of our society are proceeding along a number of parallel lines to make that shift happen.

A national movement initiated by Black women to transform the maternal health system is explicit about its demand for reproductive justice for all women of color. Eradicating bias in medical education and subsequent medical practice through textbook revision and practitioner training are key steps to transforming the system. Individualized support during the childbirth experience can also help mitigate the harms inflicted by an inattentive and biased health system. Comprehensive data collection and analysis are also being used to inform policies and practices to develop the kind of patient-centered care that Black women deserve: healthcare that is free of racial bias, promotes health equity, and improves health outcomes for Black women, other women of color, and, indeed, all birthing people. Each of these opportunities is discussed below.

Building a Movement for Reproductive Justice

Given the evidence that racism is a fundamental cause of inequities in health,[23] "improving the maternal healthcare system for all requires a commitment to anti-racism and Black women-led solutions," wrote Crear-Perry and her NBEC colleagues in 2021.[24]

The pursuit of reproductive justice had its origins in a 1994 meeting in Chicago of Black women who understood that the concerns of marginalized women, families, and communities would not be addressed by the largely middle-class and wealthy White women who were then the backbone of the most visible women's movement. Calling themselves Women of African Descent for Reproductive Justice, this group was determined to focus on the intersection of reproductive rights and social justice. SisterSong Women of Color Reproductive Justice Collective was launched three years later by 16 organizations of women from African American, Asian American, Latina, and Native American communities to build on their efforts.[25]

> Reproductive justice is "the human right to maintain personal bodily autonomy, have children, not have children, and parent the children we have in safe and sustainable communities."
>
> —SisterSong[26]

In the years that followed, other organizations emerged to advance overlapping agendas. With funding from the W.K. Kellogg Foundation, NBEC launched in New Orleans in 2015 to tackle issues related to Black infant mortality. After a convening of SisterSong and the Center for Reproductive Rights to decry the high Black maternal mortality rate, NBEC added maternal health to its mission. "The same drivers of racism, classism, and gender oppression that cause premature birth also cause maternal morbidity and mortality," said Crear-Perry. "Our goal is to undo the root causes of racism, classism, and gender oppression to ensure that all people are able to thrive."

Updating Medical Education

Medical education texts continue to impart biases about Black bodies to students, who then take those biases into practice, said Villarosa. At the same time, because most physicians are White, they come to the profession with very different lived experiences than their patients of color. Villarosa believes that medical school educators need to understand that and explicitly say, "This is something you are going to have to face and deal with and navigate and confront. We're going to teach you to do that." Today's generation of medical students gives her hope, she says, citing "activist students who are asking for a different kind of medical education, who want to be different kinds of healthcare providers, who don't want to make the same mistakes that some of their professors and predecessors made."[27]

Training Providers

As medical students move into practice, they again encounter the system's deeply embedded biases, but also witness and participate in a host of innovations designed to unpack and change them. Often, these innovations need to be evaluated and adapted to accomplish their goals. One example is the California Birth Equity Collaborative, formed in 2006 at Stanford University School of Medicine, which works with the state of California to improve birth outcomes among Black women. After implementing clinical protocols for obstetric emergencies, the number of California women who died in childbirth decreased 55% between 2006 and 2013.[28] Yet Black women remain three to four times more likely to die in childbirth than White women.

"Nothing had happened to the racial gap," said Villarosa. Recognizing that no clinical innovations have fixed racialized health disparities, the state mandated implicit bias training for anyone who works with women during pregnancy and childbirth.[29] By acknowledging and taking action against pervasive bias, California has become a model for other states.

Crear-Perry called out racism that is structural, not interpersonal, as the key factor. "If a patient's pain is not treated after having a C-section, that is not just one nurse who decides to do that. Multiple people have to be on board for that to happen, from the provider to the nurse to the pharmacy. There's a structural issue that's saying, 'we can wait on this person. Her pain is not as valuable.' Our entire structure has to be overhauled and reevaluated to think of more respectful maternity care."

A framework for doing so, built on validated measures of patient-reported experience, has been created by NBEC in partnership with the American College of Obstetrics and Gynecology, with funding from RWJF.[30] As a result, NBEC's anti-racism and birth equity trainings with maternal health providers and staff have been revamped to include helping providers learn to trust their patients. "We would never have known to do that had we not started by asking what birthing people want rather than assuming that we know what's best," Crear-Perry admitted. The Reproductive and Sexual Health Equity Framework, as it is called, has been published in the journal *Obstetrics & Gynecology*.[31] Other strategies for quality improvement, such as focused provider training, are also emerging from patient surveys and patient simulations designed to model respectful quality care.

"You're not going to get to quality improvement unless you work on undoing racism in your system," said Crear-Perry. "The gap was created by racism and will not be fixed by having the same protocols. Making everything the same and saying that's equitable doesn't acknowledge the structure of the system in the first place."

NBEC's trainings have yielded positive change, and in one Kalamazoo, Mich., hospital, the new CEO invited its board to undergo the same training. Crear-Perry saw that as a "big win" because it demonstrated that one of the hospital's highest power structures was willing to engage in confronting racism that is embedded in all parts of the organization.

Individual provider practices also need to change at every level, from the physical structure to the front desk to the clinical experience, and from the beginning of an appointment until its end.

The power dynamic in the patient–provider relationship has to change. We need to teach providers how to communicate with patients.

—Nakeitra Burse

In the value-based payment model of Healthfirst's New York City insurance plans, protocols are in place to ensure that providers tailor their treatment to meet all patient needs fully. Healthfirst providers must show that they are meeting patient-focused quality standards, and reimbursement formulas offer them incentives for providing quality care. For people of color, particularly those with limited financial means, that means offering more than medical care, said executive medical director Susan Beane. "It's also mitigating social determinant factors that can impact a person's health and well-being." (See the Spotlight at the end of this chapter.)

Provider training is an important element of Healthfirst's focus on equity, and Beane has found all providers to be very receptive, including those who do not identify themselves as persons of color. "They work together to make sure each patient receives the care they need, when they need it, from the provider who is best suited to provide it," Beane explained.

Supporting Birthing Women with Doula Care

Historically, Black women have supported each other during labor and childbirth. Indeed, Crear-Perry described having a baby as "a communal event." Today, doulas often provide some of that support as partners of pregnant, laboring, and postpartum women. These trained professionals, according to Ancient Song, an international doula certifying organization led by Black women, provide "emotional and physical support, counseling, information to make informed decisions, advocacy, and non-judgmental support" to pregnant people and their communities. Doulas are not a substitute for attentive medical care but a source of comfort and support that can reduce stress and contribute to a better birth experience. Villarosa highlighted their role as providing "a caring link to what can be a cold healthcare system."

The use of doulas has been shown to improve birth outcomes. A 2017 review of 26 studies in 17 countries found that women who received continuous one-to-one support during childbirth were more likely to have a spontaneous vaginal birth, were less likely to use pain medication or have a C-section, and had shorter labors.[32] A limitation of the findings, however, is that they did not include outcome data by race and none of the reviewed studies included low-income women.

Many obstetricians expect that their wealthy patients will have doula support, and they endorse it because the benefits are known, according to Crear-Perry. But when low-income and Black patients come with the support of a doula, "it is seen by my colleagues like they're competing with us and trying to tell us what to do," she said, still another signal of the healthcare system's racist structure. "We don't yet see this as an asset in the same way as we do for high-income patients."

Insurance coverage for doula support is limited. Doulas are not state-certified, which means that Medicaid and other insurance companies may not pay for them, although there are signs that this is changing. In Washington, D.C., an organization called Mamatoto Village offers support services through what it calls community birth workers, who assist mothers in the period that surrounds childbirth. AmeriHealth Caritas, a Medicaid-managed care plan, has partnered with Mamatoto Village to subcontract with its community birth workers to manage a population of high-risk patients. Crear-Perry believes that model can be replicated.

In 2019, New York State launched a Doula Pilot Program to study the impact of doula support on health outcomes among Medicaid recipients, according to Beane. The pilot is part of a multi-part state initiative targeting maternal mortality and racial disparities in health outcomes.

Collecting Data, Strengthening Policy, Addressing Racism

Comprehensive data are critical to understanding the extent and causes not only of maternal mortality but also of significant morbidity so that evidence-based preventive steps can be taken to substantially reduce the risks associated with pregnancy, childbirth, and their aftermath. "For every woman that dies in child-birth there are many others who almost die, who have long-term complications," stressed Crear-Perry. Looking at these cases and figuring out ways to prevent them "will be transformative."

The Maternal Mortality Review Information App system is a platform operated by the Centers for Disease Control and Prevention (CDC) to collect data on maternal mortality and morbidity. Prior to 2019, the CDC did not have the funding to fully utilize the system, so nothing more than estimates was available. Two journalistic efforts are credited with providing some of the impetus to address this gap: the 2017 National Public Radio/ProPublica special series *Lost Mothers: Maternal Mortality in the U.S.*[33] and Linda Villarosa's 2018 *New York Times Magazine* cover feature, "Why America's Black Mothers and Babies Are in a Life-or-Death Crisis."[34]

In 2018, Crear-Perry testified before Congress in support of a bill that allocated funding to the CDC to help support states in collecting rigorous maternal morbidity and mortality data. Subsequently, she and other colleagues in the reproductive justice field were part of a CDC panel that developed a data collection format that included racism and discrimination among their causes. It was an exciting moment, recalled Crear-Perry. "If you identify racism as a cause, then your review committee must talk about how it actually looks. If a patient has experienced discrimination, or if she doesn't get her pain treated or her hypertension managed in the same way, you can look at the underlying cause of racism and work to undo that."

As of July 2021, 48 states, the District of Columbia, New York City, Philadelphia, and Puerto Rico formally collect data on maternal mortality and review the reasons for each death.[35] Three examples of the impact of data:

- Burse is a member of Mississippi's Maternal Mortality Review Committee, which aims to review every maternal death in the state to identify its cause and contributing factors and to determine whether it was preventable. A licensed clinical social worker on the committee interviews the family of each deceased mother to gather the personal context. In its first report in 2019, examining deaths from 2013 through 2016, the committee made recommendations for providers, the community, and the legislature, including expanding maternal healthcare coverage to at least 12 months following a birth.[36]
- Louisiana Governor John Bel Edwards has several initiatives that address maternal and infant health. Crear-Perry sits on the Louisiana Pregnancy-Associated Mortality Review Committee, which reviewed deaths from 2011 to 2016 and issued a report in 2018.[37] The state was also the first in the Deep South to expand Medicaid, and has convened a taskforce, the Healthy Moms,

Health Babies Advisory Council, to address racial and ethnic disparities in maternal health outcomes. Still another initiative is the Louisiana Perinatal Quality Collaborative, a network of providers, public health professionals, and advocates working to promote equity and improve birth outcomes.

- Former New York Governor Andrew Cuomo established the Taskforce on Maternal Mortality and Disparate Racial Outcomes, which released its report in 2019.[38]Among its 10 recommendations was the establishment of a state-wide Maternal Mortality Review Board to study the cause of each maternal death and develop prevention strategies. Cuomo signed legislation creating the board in August 2019.[39] Other recommendations are also moving forward, according to Beane, a task force member, who expects this work to be a model for other states.

NBEC and a broad group of reproductive justice advocates have asked the Biden administration to establish a White House Office of Sexual and Reproductive Health and Well-Being. Drawing on input from the Department of Health and Human Services, the Department of Housing and Urban Development, the U.S. Agency for International Development, and other federal agencies, it would advance policies that promote wellness rather than control of women's reproductive lives.[40] In separate letters to President Joe Biden and Vice President Kamala Harris, seven U.S. senators also called on the administration to establish such an office,[41] as did 38 members of the House.[42]

Caring for Children in a Biased System

Beyond the birth and postpartum period, providing safe, nurturing, and developmentally appropriate child care is a key contributor to maternal, child, and family health and an important factor in reproductive justice. Sadly, the history and contemporary status of child care is yet another example of how bias and structural racism influence the health of Black women, both as mothers and as workers. For centuries, enslaved Black women were forced to care for the children of others, and today they are disproportionately represented in the child care workforce. Most (94%) of child-care workers are women and about 40% are women of color.[43]

The paradox of the system is that child care is unaffordable for many, while those who do the work are underpaid—some 18% of child-care workers live in poverty and qualify for public benefits, despite working full-time.[44] How we understand the work of caring for children determines how we value it, contends Shana Bartley of the Women's Law Center. Child care has been seen for centuries as a form of domestic work and, as such, has been devalued and generally relegated to people at the lowest end of the social hierarchy. "The work is very fulfilling," Bartley acknowledged, "but it is hard work. It's physically and emotionally demanding. The families you serve may be navigating many needs."

Bartley argues that child care is at least as valuable as other public goods that provide collective benefit, such as roads, schools, and fire and emergency medical services. Indeed, research evidence is clear that the first few years of life are critically important for a child's development and long-term outcomes. Reducing child care to "babysitting"—watching children to ensure they are safe—does not begin to address the benefits of quality child care that offers children opportunities for cognitive, physical, social, and emotional growth and that supports parents' return to work.

Yet the cost of child care is not spread equitably across society. "We have a mostly privatized, market-based system for something that almost everybody needs at some point and that even non-parenting people benefit from. But the system doesn't fit the value that it has in our society," said Bartley.

> *The child-care workforce is the workforce behind the workforce, the essential worker for the essential worker.*
>
> —Shana Bartley

The COVID-19 pandemic, with its many and disparate impacts on work and school routines, has hit the child-care sector especially hard.[45] For all the resulting pain, Bartley also sees an important narrative shift as society begins to recognize the real value of child care—to families, communities, and the public health infrastructure.

At the same time, she is clear that recovery will not be easy. Of the 12 million child-care slots that existed in the United States before the pandemic, at least 4.5 million will have been lost and child-care businesses will not be quick to reopen when the pandemic subsides.[46] A significant portion of the labor force is likely to be lost, with furloughed workers having moved on to other jobs, and background checks and licensing will delay efforts to fill labor gaps that are necessary to reopen.

Fewer child-care options will mean fewer women can re-enter the workforce, a blow to their economic prospects and to a broader recovery. Fewer options will also force scarcity in an already overburdened system, limiting access and becoming more expensive, which are all harmful to both maternal and child health.

An effect of the movement for Black lives and the racial reckoning triggered by events in the summer of 2020 is the acknowledgment of "the incredible work of generations of Black women in this country," stressed Bartley. She believes that it is time to construct a system that values child-care workers as skilled professionals, compensates them fairly, and treats them with respect and dignity.

She envisions a publicly financed (though not necessarily publicly run) child-care system, commenting, "Child care should not be financially inaccessible; at the same time, working in child care should not mean that you have to struggle to take care of your own family."

A Final Word

Centuries of degrading treatment, justified by a distortion of medical research and practice values and norms shaped by unexamined negative mindsets about racial inferiority, drive the inequities in the current healthcare system that damage the health of Black people today. Increasingly, healthcare providers and the system itself are showing signs that they recognize the imperative of dismantling deeply embedded practices to meet the healthcare needs of Black people in respectful and equity-informed ways.

However, *greater urgency is needed*. Black women are still losing their lives during pregnancy and childbirth and afterwards. Black infants are still dying in disproportionate numbers. The pandemic has exposed the stark reality of health inequity in a newly publicly visible way, at a time when attention to racial injustice has been heightened. A more equitable future for Black women's health and well-being is possible, and the influence of the reproductive justice movement is palpable. To meet that potential will require the sustained attention and commitment of all those who serve Black women in healthcare. The discourse has already begun.

Spotlight

Partnering to Improve Outcomes for Postpartum Women

Susan Beane, MD, Executive Medical Director, Healthfirst

Healthfirst, one of the largest not-for-profit health insurers in New York State, provides coverage for 1.6 million people through managed care plans that include Medicaid managed care, Child Health Plus, Medicare Advantage, and others. Over 40,000 providers and 80 hospitals offer services through Healthfirst plans.

As executive medical director, Dr. Susan Beane's role is to ensure that Healthfirst members achieve the best medical outcomes possible through evidence-based strategies. Her team identifies and addresses the needs of member cohorts least likely to realize these outcomes. The group also offers education to help primary care providers understand advances in evidence-based medicine and translate those advances into workable interventions.

The postpartum period offers an opportunity for high-risk new mothers to establish relationships with healthcare providers that can improve management of chronic conditions as well as their overall health and that of their children. To assess the mother's health status and initiate this care, the American College of Obstetrics and Gynecology recommends a postpartum clinical visit between 21 and 56 days after delivery. At least 80% of commercially insured mothers meet this timeline, but only about 60% of women in Medicaid managed care plans do so.[1] Transportation difficulties, child-care issues, and poor communication with providers can be barriers to completing these visits.

A partnership between Healthfirst and New York City's Mount Sinai Medical Center was designed to improve the rate at which low-income, high-risk women have a timely postpartum visit. Elizabeth A. Howell, MD, MPP, led the Mount Sinai team. "Dr. Howell and her team were very interested in whether or not some of the findings that we have had around women living in East Harlem, who are to a large extent women of color—Black and Hispanic—could achieve

Susan Beane, *Spotlight* In: *Necessary Conversations*. Edited by: Alonzo L. Plough, Oxford University Press. © Robert Wood Johnson Foundation 2022. DOI: 10.1093/oso/9780197641477.003.0007

improved outcomes with some of the evidence-based interventions that they had designed," explained Beane.

The researchers enrolled Healthfirst members who gave birth at Mount Sinai between April 2015 and October 2016 and had at least one health condition, such as hypertension, gestational diabetes, or depression.[2] A social worker and a community health worker, both conversant in English and Spanish, provided education during the postpartum hospital stay, written materials, a phone call within two weeks of delivery, and other follow-up calls as needed. Healthfirst and Mount Sinai shared the costs of the program. Public transportation costs were covered for a patient's postpartum visit, and they also received a $10 incentive to attend. Providers received small reimbursement increases for postpartum visits and participating physicians, nurses, social workers, and registrars were offered education about the visit and other clinical topics.

Compared with a control group, women who received this intervention had higher rates of both timely postpartum visits and all postpartum or gynecological visits up to 90 days following the birth. The intervention "was satisfying and relatable to a population that had demonstrable disparities in outcomes," said Beane, emphasizing the importance of the findings.

The Healthfirst team and its Mount Sinai colleagues stressed the value of the cost-sharing partnership between a Medicaid managed care plan and a health system. They positioned it as a way both to identify people at risk of less-than-optimal health outcomes and to provide them with evidence-based interventions.

Another important result of the study for Beane was that both the hospital's patient electronic health record data and the claims-based administrative data collected by the health plan showed the same outcomes. That allows the health plan to design interventions based on its own data, confident that they mirror what are found in patient records.

> *This is groundbreaking. It shows that we can trust our administrative data to demonstrate that we are achieving equity for women of color and is a foundation for doing other work like this.*
>
> —Susan Beane

The Health Harms of Incarceration and Punishment

Sherry Glied, PhD, Dean, Professor of Public Service, Robert F. Wagner Graduate School of Public Service, New York University

Alesha Judkins, Mississippi State Director, Criminal Justice Reform, FWD.us

Rukia Lumumba, JD, Founding Executive Director, People's Advocacy Institute and Electoral Justice CoDirector, Movement for Black Lives

Faced with a growing body of health evidence about the damage inflicted by mass incarceration and a widening lens on what it means to be marginalized, RWJF officially embraced incarceration as a social determinant of health and well-being in 2018, adding it to the 35 national-level measures it uses to track the nation's progress toward achieving well-being and health equity.[1]

The United States incarcerates a higher percentage of its population than any other nation in the world,[2] making mass incarceration and the disproportionate number of incarcerated people of color arguably one of the most pressing civil rights issues in the United States today. Highlighted by a pandemic that did its greatest harm to people of color and intensified economic disparities, structural racism in the criminal justice and carceral systems and a pattern of unjust police killings of Black people have finally earned the nation's attention.

Nevertheless, if awareness of the detrimental effects of mass incarceration has been growing, the impact of imprisonment and punishment on health and health disparities has received much less attention. Study after study have demonstrated the clear facts: Incarceration and health are deeply interrelated, not only for those who reside in jails and prisons, but also for their families, their communities, and the nation as a whole.[3]

Sherry Glied, Alesha Judkins, and Rukia Lumumba, *The Health Harms of Incarceration and Punishment* In: *Necessary Conversations*. Edited by: Alonzo L. Plough, Oxford University Press. © Robert Wood Johnson Foundation 2022.
DOI: 10.1093/oso/9780197641477.003.0008

This chapter documents how and why the nation's incarceration problem is not only a justice problem—it is also a health problem. After a brief statistical review, NYU/Wagner's Sherry Glied offers a dire health profile of those who cycle through prisons and jails. Alesha Judkins from FWD.us discusses what she calls an "incarceration crisis" in Mississippi, where long prison sentences have become the norm. Rukia Lumumba of People's Advocacy Institute (PAI) explains that the health impacts of the criminal justice system begin long before an individual first comes into contact with law enforcement and continue through incarceration and reentry. The three contributors also identify opportunities to reverse incarceration trends, highlighting the role of education and early intervention, and the need to address the root causes of the health disparities that arise when society sends too many people to prison for too long.

Structural Racism: Incarceration by the Numbers

At least 4.9 million people are arrested and incarcerated each year in the United States.[4] According to RWJF's 2019 study on mass incarceration's threat to health equity, an estimated 2.2 million adults are in prison or jail on any given day, and more than 45,000 youth are in juvenile detention facilities, adult prisons, and jails.[5] Prisons are institutions under state or federal jurisdiction that confine people convicted of serious crimes, while jails are operated under local governments to confine people awaiting trial or punish those convicted of minor crimes. Juvenile detention is primarily for youths accused of committing crimes at age 18 or younger, although age cutoffs vary by state and teenagers are sometimes punished as adults.

To a degree, these numbers reflected a promising trend: After a steady rise every year from 1980 to 2008, the number of people imprisoned on a daily basis in the United States has decreased to its lowest level in more than two decades. And while rates declined across racial and ethnic groups, "the greatest decline has come among Black Americans, whose imprisonment rate has decreased 34% since 2006."[6] This compares to a decline of 26% among Hispanics and 17% among Whites.

But the data remain grim. Every day, more than half a million adults who have not been sentenced or convicted of any crime remain in U.S. jails simply because they cannot afford to pay the bail required to secure their release. These adults account for nearly all of the jail population growth between 1997 and 2017.[7] And as the RWJF report pointed out, "Both the number of people incarcerated and the incarceration rate in the United States still exceed those of every other nation in the world, including totalitarian regimes. This unacceptable level of incarceration—often referred to as mass incarceration—appears to be the result of policies engaged from the 1970s through the 1990s that imposed tougher penalties for crimes, including more severe sentencing and compulsory incarceration for minor repeat offenses."[8]

These discriminatory policies included the so-called war on drugs and the Anti-Drug Abuse Act of the 1980s, which used incarceration to respond to addiction and drug use in Black populations; the 1994 federal "three-strikes" provision that mandated life sentences for offenders convicted of a violent crime after two or more prior convictions, even for nonviolent crimes, such as a drug offense; and more recent policing practices, such as New York City's "stop-and-frisk" strategy that largely targeted young Black men.[9]

The decline in incarcerated Black Americans, while real, does not mask the reality that the numbers remain staggeringly disproportionate. The Black imprisonment rate (1,501 incarcerated individuals for every 100,000 Black adults) is nearly twice the rate of Hispanics (797 per 100,000) and more than five times the rate among Whites (268 per 100,000).[10] By 2020, Black and Brown people made up 60% of those incarcerated in the United States, though they represented 39% of the population nationally.[11]

> *The United States incarcerates many more persons—both in absolute numbers and as a percentage of the population—than any other nation in the world.*—RWJF report, *Mass Incarceration Threatens Health Equity in America*

The 30,000-Foot Perspective

Economist and policy researcher Sherry Glied acknowledges that she looks at the world from what is essentially an airplane window. She recently assumed this airborne "30,000-foot perspective" to examine incarceration and its relationship with health through Medicaid data collected from individuals who have been incarcerated on Rikers Island.

While it is eventually slated to close, Rikers remains the largest correctional facility in New York City, housing up to 9,000 people a day. Called one of "America's 10 worst prisons," it is notorious for violence, staff brutality, and abuse of adolescents, and features one of the nation's highest rates of solitary confinement and unconscionably long periods of detention for those who cannot make bail.[12] The horrific realities of Rikers were made visible in the tragic story of Kalief Browder, a Black Bronx high school student who spent three years in Rikers (two in solitary confinement) because his family could not afford his $3,000 bail. Browder, accused of stealing a backpack but never convicted of a crime, died by suicide in 2015, two years after he was finally released.

Glied set out to describe the health, healthcare utilization patterns, and healthcare expenditures of people involved in the New York City criminal justice system. Her study drew on five years of New York State Medicaid data for over 6 million enrollees and was conducted under the auspices of RWJF's Policies for Action, a research program that conducts policy and law research to build a Culture of Health. Mining the data from 2012 to 2016, she identified nearly 70,000 people who had been released from Rikers, two-thirds of whom had Medicaid claims after being discharged.

Digging deeper into the data, she uncovered a subset population that had cycled through Rikers six times or more since 2012. Glied soon realized that these high utilizers, representing 10% of her study population, were the exact population she needed to study.

The Health Profile of High Utilizers

Research has shown that rates of communicable diseases, chronic health conditions, and psychiatric and substance use disorders are significantly higher among individuals who have been incarcerated than among those who have not been.[13]

> *Any amount of jail is associated with a higher prevalence of chronic health conditions. They're just sicker than everybody else.*
>
> —Sherry Glied

Glied quickly confirmed that, as is the case everywhere in the United States, incarcerated high utilizers in New York are disproportionately people of color: 57% are Black (though the city's population is about 24% Black) and 31% are Latino, 89% are male, and their average age is 35. The vast majority are jailed for misdemeanors. She calculated that high utilizers at Rikers "spent nearly a year in jail over that five-year period, although they were never there for very long at any one time."

In collaboration with several city agencies, Glied used the extensive Medicaid data to ask a very specific question: What are the health correlates of repeated incarceration on high utilizers, compared to those of people who are incarcerated at Rikers only once? She soon had answers:[14]

- Those repeatedly incarcerated had much higher rates of cardiovascular disease, liver disease, asthma, hypertension, and diabetes than other people of similar race, age, and gender in the Medicaid data.
- When compared to people who are in jail only once, people sent back to jail over and over are 25% more likely to have a serious health condition, and the

rate at which they have these health conditions is remarkably high: Over one-third of the population had diabetes, one-fourth had cardiovascular disease, and they were about twice as likely to have a serious mental illness.

- The biggest health problem among high utilizers is chronic alcohol or substance use, diagnosed after they leave jail. Nearly 65% of high utilizers had an admission or a diagnosis of an alcohol or substance use problem during a medical visit in the five years studied, compared to 46% of those with one jail visit.

- Those who cycle in and out of Rikers were twice as likely to have an inpatient hospitalization compared to those who were jailed only once, with about three-quarters of those inpatient hospitalizations for alcohol or substance use disorders. Glied said she was "really stunned by the extremely high rates of substance use and alcohol use that are comorbid with the mental health conditions."

Glied's study also found that a very small number of people account for a great deal of the resource utilization.[15] New York City officials, Glied noted, were not only spending money repeatedly jailing individuals but then spent nearly double the Medicaid dollars on high utilizers after they were discharged, compared to what they typically spent on people who had been jailed only once.

"There's a lot of money on the table here, particularly for people with alcohol and substance use problems. We are keeping them in jail—or keeping them in hospitals," said Glied. Once she pointed this out, Glied noticed that city health and policy officials began to consider what services they should provide outside jail to prevent their return. Said Glied: "We're going to have to make a very specific intervention in one of these systems, and this 30,000-foot methodology helps us get at what we in economics call the 'causal inference:' Which of these things actually causes health outcomes to be worse? And that's the one we will try to reform first."

Glied is quick to note that the study provides unique insights into how the justice system reflects and perpetuates the "fundamental flaws and the evils of structural racism and inequality of American society."

"The justice system is embedded in a society that has those flaws, and so is the healthcare system," she emphasized. "We're talking about two sets of mechanisms, two sets of processes that are happening in parallel. That's actually a methodological complexity we need to understand as we come to think about the role of reform. Because that's at the heart of the problem when trying to think about policy reform in the justice field in a way that improves health: How do we keep it from perpetuating society's flaws?"

The population that comes out of jail is not only impacted by their experi-ence of being in jail. They're also coming from and going into a society that is deeply unequal and has a lot of problems with it. This is not a healthy way to have a society.

—Sherry Glied

Incarceration in Mississippi

Although New York City and Jackson, Miss., are vastly differently places, Glied believes that "they share a lot of the same pathologies that infect all of American life." Certainly, the pathologies of racial discrimination and health inequity are parallel. Alesha Judkins sees them every day in her work as Mississippi State Director of Criminal Justice Reform for FWD.us, a policy advocacy group that targets injustice in the carceral system throughout the state.

Where Glied's viewpoint of what goes on in prisons is expansive and data-driven, Judkins has a more personal lens. She has been an eyewitness to the abysmal conditions inside Mississippi state prisons, which house over 652 people for every 100,000 Mississippians, the second highest rate of imprison-ment in the United States, behind Louisiana. The Black men who make up 13% of the state's residents account for 75% of those serving 20-plus-year prison sentences.[16]

Acknowledging an "incarceration crisis in Mississippi," Judkins described the conditions she has seen or heard about in multiple prisons during her 10 years working for incarceration justice throughout the state and inside the 4,800-bed Mississippi State Penitentiary. Commonly known as Parchman Farm, it was once a 17,000-acre plantation and is now a maximum-security prison located in a poor, rural Mississippi Delta community. Incarceration conditions there and elsewhere almost defy belief, and certainly they defy humanity.

According to Judkins, 24 deaths occurred in Mississippi prisons in January and February 2020 alone. "Yes, you heard me correctly: 24 deaths," she reiterated. To draw attention to the system's unsafe conditions, incarcerated people had recently attracted national headlines by using cellphones to send out pictures and videos of their grueling circumstances. Judson recounted both re-cent and past horror stories, including that of a man serving a five-year sentence who went blind after being denied his glaucoma medicine; an incarcerated indi-vidual placed in solitary confinement for "acting out," when the real issue was his untreated high blood sugar; a diabetic individual, with open leg and ankle sores from shackles on his bare skin, whose nurse pleaded with officers not to put him in leg irons, knowing he was at risk of having his leg amputated.

Mississippi's extreme and habitual sentencing laws impose harsh sentences on people convicted of first felonies and stack sentences on top of one another—Judkins described how a person convicted of a first-time drug possession can be sentenced to 20 years in prison and how a person with a third drug offense can serve 60 mandatory years. A high-profile lawsuit on behalf of more than 150 incarcerated individuals demanded that Parchman be closed, accusing the Mississippi Department of Corrections of gross negligence and alleging "barbaric" conditions that included food contaminated with rat feces and cockroaches, flooded cells, toxic black mold, and sweltering heat. A lack of beds meant some people were sleeping on floors, and medical and mental health resources were utterly inadequate.[17]

Judkins's portrait was nearly impossible to visualize. As the enormity of the state's incarceration crisis sunk in, a member of the *Sharing Knowledge* conference where she made her presentation asked a moving question: "When your work every day is witnessing, observing, absorbing all the pain and suffering you are describing, I wonder: 'How do you get up in the morning?'"

Judkins was ready with an answer. "The years of relationships I've built with men who are incarcerated—who I know are counting on me—that fuels me," said Judkins, who has worked with clients on death row, investigated unconstitutional living conditions, and helped lead bail reform efforts during her career in transformative justice work. "So if they can have hope in this situation that they're living in, I've got to put on my big girl pants and keep going."

> When you think of what happens in poor and rural communities when it comes to lack of healthcare and the impact of racial discrimination, just magnify that times 10 for our prison communities and what they have to endure and suffer.
>
> —Alesha Judkins

Three Friends, Sentenced for Life

Like Judkins, attorney and human rights activist Rukia Lumumba knows that racism and inequities in the carceral system harm people of color long before[18] and long after their arrests.[19] Growing up in Jackson as the daughter of civil rights activists, her father was renowned human rights activist, lawyer, and former Jackson Mayor Chokwe Lumumba, who was repeatedly thrown in jail for being in contempt of court as he "zealously represented his clients," she recalled. Though the seeds of activism were planted early, what ultimately led Lumumba to a career devoted to transformative justice was the experiences of high school classmates who began serving life sentences in prison while she was a college freshman.

One friend, Azikiwe Kambule, 15, "spent his entire adolescence and young adulthood in prison," she noted, after being wrongfully charged and convicted of armed carjacking and an accessory to the murder of a Jackson school-teacher. With the help of Amnesty International, his case was overturned when he was 30 and he eventually returned to South Africa where his family had relocated.

Terun Moore—another friend "who was like a little brother, I would take him to school every morning"—was charged with murder and sentenced as a teen-ager to life without parole, although records show that he acted in self-defense. After serving 19 years in adult confinement, he was paroled in 2017, with the help of the Southern Poverty Law Center, which had long advocated for the re-lease of youths charged as adults.

Upon release, Moore helped Lumumba co-found the PAI, which focuses on three areas: electoral justice and making sure incarcerated individuals have the right to vote; providing legal support for those serving long and life sentences and helping families secure their release; and community capacity building, which includes serving as an incubator for bail fund projects, prison reform coalitions, and violence interruption programs. Together, Moore and Lumumba are trying to obtain parole release for her third childhood friend, who Lumumba said "received a grossly punitive sentence" after being convicted on drug and drug trafficking charges and is still behind bars.

How Punishment Triggers Health Inequities

The stories of her three friends illustrate why Lumumba distinguishes between "incarceration" and "punishment" as she describes how health harms and inequi-ties start.

To Lumumba, incarceration is a word that people recognize and to which they respond in different ways—"it runs the spectrum of folks thinking 'we incar-cerate too many' or 'people deserve to do the time for the crime,'" she said. But in her view, incarceration is not the place where health inequities in the carceral system begin. Rather, she argues, there is an impact on health the moment there is a threat of punishment. Punishment, she says, is inflicted when a Black man or woman is profiled or questioned—on the way to school, walking down the street or into a store, pulled over at a traffic stop. Punishment is when someone is incarcerated and denied water or medication. Punishment is getting out of prison with deteriorated health and facing a stigma so great that, in places like Mississippi, state policies and practices make it impossible to receive adequate health insurance, including state-provided Medicaid coverage or adequate food voucher and housing subsidies because of your criminal history.

The very first engagement with the carceral system can trigger cascading layers of prejudicial treatment that increase a person's risks of poor health and undermine health equity for individuals, families, and communities alike.[20] Consider these vicious cycles:

- Discriminatory treatment by both the police and the courts markedly heightens the likelihood of incarceration among people of color and poor people in all racial groups. The experience of being jailed or imprisoned then leads to worse health, linked to unhealthy conditions during incarceration (overcrowding, violence, sexual and physical abuse, and poor sanitation) and after release (social exclusion and marginalization, reflected in barriers to employment and earnings potential).
- Social exclusion and marginalization after incarceration, in turn, lead to greater poverty, powerlessness, and homelessness, further exacerbating the risks of poor health. A similar impact can occur even if a person is not incarcerated: For example, racism and prejudicial treatment by police can lead to ill health indirectly, through the physiological consequences of stress, or directly, if the police use excessive force.
- A household member's incarceration can have drastic consequences for a family's health and well-being: An estimated 2.7 million children nationwide are growing up with one or both parents behind bars, while approximately 10 million children have experienced parental incarceration at some point in their lives. Parental incarceration increases children's risk of drug abuse, criminality, and delinquency as they mature and predicts a wide range of health problems.
- According to the ACLU, the "school-to-prison pipeline"—a disturbing national trend in which children are funneled out of public schools and into disciplinary alternative schools or the juvenile justice system—primarily affects children with histories of poverty, abuse, neglect, or learning disabilities who would benefit from supportive educational and counseling services, not isolation and punishment. This trend has escalated as more schools adopt zero-tolerance policies that criminalize minor infractions and employ police officers, rather than centering resources and trained personnel on challenges that can be addressed within the educational setting.[21]

When Lumumba considers where health inequities begin, she thinks not only about her three childhood friends but about one 15-year-old—a student she met while representing young people and establishing alternatives-to-incarceration programs in New York City for 10 years early in her career. "On his way to school every day, he was stopped by police four times—literally *four times* on his way to school. And then once he got to school, he was searched through metal detectors. And he wasn't an exception to the rule—this was pretty much what happened to most of the children I worked with."

This memory drives her. "What does that do to your psyche, to your ability to protect yourself, to your right to privacy and personhood? I have heard teenagers normalize these frequent stops and frisks, as if they have no power or autonomy over what happens to their bodies, their future, or their ability to remain free of incarceration. They are consistently faced with the fear of being locked up daily. It begins to limit your ability to think and dream a little bigger and outside of the bounds. And that's punishment—mental punishment—and it impacts our mental health and our lives long before we even know it."

> *Punishment leaves us at a place where all we're doing is causing more harm to someone else. We're not helping to relieve the pain and heal—we're creating more pain.*
>
> —Rukia Lumumba

What Can Be Done?

There is a way forward, Lumumba insisted, a way "to move [from] a system of punishment to one that's more transformative, that doesn't have as many disparate health impacts." Directing her questions to Sherry Glied and Alesha Judkins, who shared the stage with her on a *Sharing Knowledge* panel, Lumumba asked: What solutions do you believe will help decrease disparate health outcomes on people who are involved in the criminal system?

- Glied described three ongoing studies using Medicaid data to learn more about health outcomes by answering these questions:
  o What is the relationship between Medicaid enrollment and jail recidivism? For those with alcohol and substance use issues before incarceration, can you determine if problems for families and individuals intensified prior to incarceration?
  o Do residents of neighborhoods with higher incidence of stop and frisk see greater mental health benefits when this policy ends?
  o Does a recent change in New York City's Medicaid policy that allows people to connect more quickly with Medicaid services help interrupt the cycle of repeat utilization?

- Judkins and Lumumba highlighted a number of initiatives within their organizations to address key inequities within the carceral system: putting an end to cash bail, a practice that primarily keeps poor people in jail and disproportionately impacts Black and Latino people who are awaiting trial; reducing extreme sentencing and ending habitual sentencing in places like Mississippi; securing release for more adults unfairly incarcerated and those charged as youths; ending mass incarceration; working to close Parchman; and investing savings from the criminal justice system back into communities.

- Judkins also emphasized the importance of restoring families impacted by incarceration. "Ripping people from their families" by sending them to prisons two or three hours away from home requires those left behind to pay for transportation, take time off from work to visit, and shoulder exorbitant costs to receive telephone calls from inside prisons. "You take away the only kind of connection of love and family that you have, and that negatively impacts everyone's health. Just restore families by enacting policies that are going to get people back home."

- Judkins and Glied both argued that educational systems can provide early interventions to keep young people in school and out of the criminal justice system. Harkening back to her early years as a teacher, Judkins stressed the need to understand what is happening in the lives of at-risk students who act out: Is he hungry? Is she being bullied? What is going on at home that led to this behavior? The answers might suggest interventions that are supportive rather than punitive.

- Glied drew a direct line between keeping families out of poverty and being able to live a life free of the carceral system. "There is a growing body of literature showing that making investments in families and children—with housing, education, direct financial support services, food—is really good for kids and it keeps them out of prison and jail when they get older," Glied said. "There really are opportunities for doing better before this whole cycle escalates."

In closing, Lumumba echoed a message heard throughout the conference: Solutions to problems and greater health equity can best be found through those "closest to the pain. Community is central, not peripheral, to equity," she said. "Individuals, grassroots groups, faith and neighborhood organizations in local communities are most effective in doing work that is transformational."

Lumumba pointed out that within the PAI, an incubator program called Strong Arms of JXN uses a "credible messenger" approach to train, mentor, and provide resources to people hardest hit by mass incarceration. The program, which involves local people whose lived experience is similar to those they are mentoring, is part of PAI's Violence Interruption Initiative. That work also includes a community evaluation of police and community education efforts to stop violence by building community resources and understanding.

> *Accountability is actually what we should be striving towards. We have to have investment in communities, and it can't just be on the back of foundation dollars. It has to be integral to the government of that place.*
>
> —Rukia Lumumba

COVID-19 and Incarceration

There was one approaching incarceration inequity that Lumumba, Glied, and Judkins could not have anticipated during the *Sharing Knowledge* conference: The health disparities in prisons that were tragically magnified when COVID-19 hit.

By the end of 2020, more than 570,000 residents of U.S. jails and prisons (nearly one in five incarcerated individuals) had contracted the coronavirus over the past year, and at least 2,500 residents and staff had died.[22] By April 2021, in a special report that tracked every known coronavirus case in every correctional setting in the United States (including state and federal prisons, immigrant detention centers, juvenile detention facilities, and county and regional jails), the *New York Times* reported that "America's prisons, jails, and detention centers have been among the nation's most dangerous places when it comes to infections from the coronavirus. Over the past year, more than 1,400 new inmate infections and seven deaths, on average, have been reported inside those facilities each day."[23]

According to Judkins, incarcerated people in Mississippi prisons are incredibly likely to be infected by COVID-19 and bold, immediate action is needed by state leaders to reduce the prison population.

In Philadelphia, where the city's COVID-19 "shelter-in-place" policy required incarcerated people to stay in their cells for nearly 24 hours a day, the extreme lockdown measures had dire consequences for both mental and physical health: Suicide attempts per capita doubled compared with prior years, and three people were killed in city jails in six months, a rate considered 15 times higher than the national average.[24]

In a December 2020 episode of "Ear Hustle," a podcast made and produced by incarcerated individuals at San Quentin State Prison in the San Francisco Bay area, a man described the experience of being locked down, lacking the basic resources of fresh air, soap, and water to fight a virus he could not see, and knowing that more than 100 incarcerated men had already died from it:[25]

I have to sit here and wait for my death to come. And the truth was, we were never as scared or as uncertain as when COVID started taking people out. This was the only time we were really like, "We are going to die. And we can't escape it."

—Incarcerated individual, San Quentin

As the pandemic moved into its second year, the statistics on incarcerated individuals were not encouraging.

Around the country, prisons and jails that had initially managed to reduce their populations to limit the spread of disease were again nearing capacity limits, defying the public sentiment reflected in national polls: "Voters nation-wide supported releasing people from jails and prisons as a means of containing the spread of COVID-19 and protecting public health."[26] A comparison of pa-role rates in 13 states by the Prison Policy Initiative showed that parole boards approved fewer releases in 2020 than in the previous year, "despite the raging pandemic."[27] A scathing report on so-called progressive prosecutors pointed out that many had failed to make long-promised changes to alter mass incarceration at a time when "we need to reduce our jail and prison populations by 80% for the United States to even look similar to other comparable nations."[28]

In Mississippi, FWD.us reported that 106 incarcerated people had died in state prisons from late December 2019 to the end of 2020; at least 28 more died in the first six months of 2021.[29] According to the report, "The consequences of not passing criminal justice reform last legislative season have been deadly."[30]

Moving Forward, Step by Step

Despite the health inequities underscored by COVID-19, the early months of 2021 saw a few promising steps toward incarceration reform with the potential to reduce the degree of contact people have with the justice system.

In line with broader national trends, Florida voters approved a referendum giving many formerly incarcerated felons the right to vote (although the state subsequently took action that weakened that decision[31]). The movement to eliminate cash bail progressed across the country, with Illinois becoming the first state to end it entirely.[32] In his first week as president, Joe Biden issued four executive orders designed to advance "the state of equity" in the criminal justice system and the Department of Justice.[33] Although his orders did not specifically address the high number of incarcerated people, they highlighted the need to reduce profit-based incentives to put people in prison by phasing out privately operated criminal detention facilities.

The Mississippi state legislature moved in February 2021 to advance two bills that finally addressed the state's dangerously high prison population by reducing its harsh and habitual sentencing requirements. While noting that the current draft of bills did "not go far enough," a nonetheless relieved Judkins acknowledged that they represented significant progress.[34]

And in April 2021, the Mississippi state legislature took what Judkins called "courageous steps to begin addressing a worsening prison crisis" when it passed a bill that significantly expanded parole eligibility in the state.[35] Before the bill was signed into law, Judkins noted that only one-third of the prison population was eligible for a parole hearing. "Now," she said, "two-thirds of the prison population will have the opportunity to go before the parole board for the opportunity to be reunited with their families and communities."

> *These much-needed reforms will make prisons safer, reduce wasteful taxpayer spending, and restore hope to thousands of Mississippians and their families.*
>
> —Alesha Judkins

In a seminal year of steps both backward and forward, the importance of redistributing resources where they do the most good was reflected in the cry to "defund the police." That demand is closely tied to the abolitionist movement, which argues that the $182 billion spent each year by local, state, and federal governments on corrections, policing, and criminal court systems[36] could be better allocated to housing, education, health, employment, and community resources for marginalized and disenfranchised populations.

That message is echoed by the abolitionist coalition Movement for Black Lives and from well-known abolitionist leaders like Angela Davis and activist/scholar Ruth Wilson Gilmore. Responding to renewed calls for action and echoing RWJF's view of mass incarceration as a social determinant of health, a new generation of abolitionist activists have embraced Gilmore's core message that "abolition" means more than closing prisons; it means embracing the need for and creating "vital systems of support that many communities lack. Abolitionists ask how we resolve inequalities and get people the resources they need long before they 'mess up.'"[37]

As Lumumba concluded, "It's actually about reinvesting in community, by taking dollars away from institutions of policing that have not helped to effectively reduce violence or harm. Defund the Police is not about taking people's jobs; it is actually protecting people's lives."

We need to ensure that we are so invested in community that institutions of policing are either no longer necessary or they have shifted to being totally about the well-being of a community.

—Rukia Lumumba

A Final Word

In its report on how mass incarceration threatens health equity, RWJF insisted that the debate over mass incarceration had gone on long enough and declared, "We know enough to act." The report concluded, "We have a choice as a society. We can continue to approach crime and punishment in ways that violate our values and drain immense levels of government resources, or we can redirect our efforts away from mass incarceration—choosing instead to focus on treatment, rehabilitation, and providing equitable opportunities for every American to live a dignified and healthy life free of unjust, inhumane, and unnecessary incarceration."[38]

Our central aim at the Robert Wood Johnson Foundation is the achievement of health equity. And we know we can't reach that goal unless, as a nation, we address mass incarceration.
—RWJF report, *Mass Incarceration Threatens Health Equity in America*

Immigrant Health

Inequity and Fear

Mark Hall, JD, Director of Health Law and Policy Program, Professor of Law, Wake Forest University

Alana M.W. LeBrón, PhD, Assistant Professor, Department of Health, Society, and Behavior, Program in Public Health and Department of Chicano/Latino Studies, School of Social Sciences, University of California, Irvine

Milena A. Melo, PhD, Assistant Professor, Department of Anthropology, University of Texas Rio Grande Valley

Julie Morita, MD, Executive Vice President, Robert Wood Johnson Foundation

Mariana Osoria, MA, Senior Vice President, Partnerships & Engagement, Family Focus

Very little so fully distorts the ways in which people who reside in the United States see one another—or so completely undermines the quest for racial justice—than the use of this phrase: illegal immigrant.

In a conversation focused on immigrant health, inequity, and fear, Alana LeBrón, assistant professor at the University of California, Irvine, set down a single ground rule at the *Sharing Knowledge* session she was moderating: No one should speak those words. She invited everyone to recognize that being undocumented or having an "unauthorized" presence are "social constructs that attempt to define who belongs in a given society and represent a critical form of structural racism." She implored everyone to never "dehumanize people when using language."

Mark Hall, Alana M.W. LeBrón, Milena A. Melo, Julie Morita, and Mariana Osoria, *Immigrant Health* In: *Necessary Conversations*. Edited by: Alonzo L. Plough, Oxford University Press. © Robert Wood Johnson Foundation 2022. DOI: 10.1093/oso/9780197641477.003.0009

"As we explore the immigrant and migrant experience, and the connection between immigration laws and policies and implications for health, I want to acknowledge that no human being is illegal," said LeBrón. And then, for emphasis, she said it again.

> *As immigrant rights advocates have long asserted, no human being is illegal.*
> —Alana LeBrón

In this chapter, contributors review the impact of structural inequity and fear on immigrant health. LeBrón is joined by Mark Hall of Wake Forest University, the University of Texas Rio Grande Valley's Milena Melo, RWJF's Julie Morita, and Mariana Osoria from Family Focus to discuss how the health of immigrants and the health of their communities are impacted by racism, inequities, and fear of participating in civic life—especially when people risk being deported and separated from their families.

Along with research and data, the contributors offer poignant, personal stories of what it means to live with increased surveillance in Texas along the Mexican border, how immigration policies keep people from essential health programs in Illinois, and what the fear of being observed in even ordinary activities does to health in North Carolina. The contributors also consider the disproportionate impact of COVID-19 on immigrant communities and review opportunities to change what Morita called "the false and damaging narratives of racial hierarchy in America."

> *We need to concentrate on policies that shift power and give voice and agency to people who face the most pernicious barriers to well-being.*
> —Julie Morita

Contemporary Anti-Immigration Policies

Since 1965, when U.S. immigration laws replaced a national quota system, the number of immigrants living in this country has more than quadrupled to nearly 13.7% of the population (still below the record 14.8% immigrant population share recorded in 1890).[1] Over the last several decades—and across Democratic and Republican administrations—the nation has struggled with competing views about immigration and immigrants, failed to consider the full context of the issues involved, and witnessed an unprecedented rise in anti-immigration policies.[2]

The country's 10.5 million undocumented immigrants, who are in this country without a recognized legal status, have been particularly affected. In

2018, they represented 23% of the 44.8 million U.S. residents born outside the country.[3] While the number of undocumented Mexican immigrants has fallen by 2 million since its peak of 6.7 million in 2007—and they now represent less than half of the country's undocumented immigrant population—undocumented immigrants from other parts of the world increased from 2007 to 2017, especially regions in Asia and Central America.[4]

A primary feature of immigrant communities is mixed-status families whose members may include a mix of undocumented people, U.S. citizens, permanent residents, and those with temporary statuses, including the Deferred Action for Childhood Arrivals (DACA), which has sheltered hundreds of thousands of undocumented youths from deportation. There are approximately 2.3 million mixed-status families in the United States, according to a study by former DACA recipient Milena Melo,[5] a situation, she says, that "is largely the result of the decline in opportunities to regularize legal status over the last two decades as well as increased border militarization that has made it more difficult for people to circulate between the U.S. and their home country."[6]

> It's hard to not know someone who is undocumented or who has DACA. So when you're talking about policies affecting undocumented immigrants, it's affecting entire families, entire communities, and even a lot of people who are U.S. citizens. Entire families are vulnerable.
>
> —Milena Melo

Racism and Inequity: Bad for the Nation's Soul and Health Status

The rising threat to immigrant households in recent decades has raised significant concerns about the health consequences of immigration policy, the threat of deportation, and the structural racism that is often the unspoken foundation of stringent immigration enforcement. According to Melo, "They're so intertwined that you can't really talk about immigration without talking about racism, right?"

The story of immigration in this country carries a harsh reality: These stories are not created equal. As reported by the Center for Health Progress, "White immigrants have historically been provided certain rights and privileges, like citizenship status or the ability to own land. Immigrants of color, on the other hand, have faced blatant persecution . . . While immigrants of all statuses, ethnicities, and backgrounds are seemingly under attack these days, it's also clear that some immigrants are being attacked more than others."[7] Some recent examples, the Center reported, include Latino parents being separated from their children;

immigrants from predominately Muslim countries being banned from the United States; the escalating rates of deportation of immigrants from African countries and immigrants of African descent, such as Haitian people; and a previous administration that "repeatedly lashed out against immigrants of color, calling Mexican immigrants 'animals.'" Another report noted that the 1.7 million undocumented Asian Americans and Pacific Islanders in the United States are five times more likely to be deported for criminal convictions than other immigrant groups and, more specifically, that Southeast Asians and Pacific Islanders are deported at a rate of three times more than that of immigrants as a whole.[8]

Understanding how structural racism is embedded in immigration policies and influences the lives of undocumented immigrants and their families and communities provides the evidence that can drive change. Ongoing research into these areas, said Julie Morita, provides irrefutable proof that deep-rooted barriers to health and discrimination have profound impacts on the health of immigrant communities.

> *Racism has its own virulence that is bad for the nation's soul and, as research has shown, is actually bad for the nation's health.*[9]
>
> —Julie Morita

Immigration and Health

Citing study after study, the *Sharing Knowledge* contributors point to evidence that unstable immigration status leads to poorer physical and mental health outcomes for adults and children alike. The contributors were particularly focused on the implications for Latino communities.

Less Likely to Seek Health Treatment

When people feel threatened, fearful or distrustful, they are less likely to seek health treatment or engage with the medical, law enforcement, and social services systems. In his study of Latino immigrants, researcher Mark Hall "found that various anti-immigrant laws and policies have a chilling effect on the use of needed health and other services, as well as access to basic utilities, healthy foods, and public spaces for recreation and physical activity." Hall is an expert in healthcare law and public policy at Wake Forest University and an RWJF *Investigator Awards in Health Policy* recipient.

He noted that these detrimental impacts are particularly acute for children and young people, as "immigrant parents face difficult decisions about whether to access services for their children and potentially risk exposure to immigration enforcement." He highlighted two policies with particularly severe consequences.

One was the fear and confusion caused by changes to the federal "public charge" rule, which required applicants for permanent residency status to prove they will not primarily rely on government benefits, such as financial assistance, food programs, or Medicaid. Hall said a harsher version of the public charge rule adopted in 2019 "had a demonstrably negative impact by deterring immigrant families from seeking a range of legitimate public health and social support services, especially for children." (That rule was vacated by the courts in November 2020 and is no longer in effect.[10])

The other chilling policy, known as the 287(g) program, allows state and local authorities to essentially be deputized as immigration enforcers, raising the risk that even local traffic stops will lead to legal action.[11] After 287(g) was implemented in North Carolina, Hall and his colleagues documented a long list of troubling health effects stemming from distrust of systems, lack of access to providers, risky self-care, and transportation barriers exacerbated by the fear of traffic stops. The results were inadequate prenatal care, delays in receiving preventive services or medical treatment, profoundly compromised child health, and increased mental health challenges.[12]

Mental and Physical Health Harms from Heightened Surveillance

Heightened rates and threats of deportation, immigration surveillance, restrictive immigrant policies, and racialized policing harm the mental and physical health of Latino populations. According to a study by LeBrón and colleagues called "Policing Us Sick,"[13] restrictive immigration policies and deportations under the Secure Communities program—a coordinated effort by federal and local law enforcement to identify, detain, and deport immigrants without authorized U.S. status—increase the mental health needs of Latino populations. Both the threat of deportation and knowing someone who has been deported correlate with poorer mental health. Likewise, according to the study, "Latinos who reported that 'people like me' are more likely to be stopped by police, arrested, or sent to prison were more likely than their counterparts to report poor physical health."

"We have seen that immigrants and immigrant communities are often under unrelenting pressure to carefully assess their circumstances, reduce risk, and avert the gaze of governmental institutions," said LeBrón. "The consequences of these coping responses are reflected in mistrust of public health institutions, healthcare systems, and police, documented declines in cardiovascular health and mental health, and an increased risk of adverse birth outcomes, to name a few."

Zeroing in on women of Mexican origin living in Detroit, LeBrón reported similar health consequences. As she noted in a report called "They Are Clipping Our Wings,"[14] restrictive immigrant policies directed at someone because of a legal status that is known or assumed, or based on appearance or language spoken, acutely affect social conditions, increase economic vulnerability, and limit access to health-related resources. Such policies are often accompanied by anti-immigrant sentiments and have an impact that reverberates across generations, social networks, and legal status.

"A few women described these systems of racism as 'clipping their wings' or making them 'feel like a caged bird,'" LeBrón wrote. For example, the lack of a driver's license or an official state identification can make shopping, doctor's visits, or other routine errands more difficult, forcing people to become hypervigilant in order to avoid encounters with police and immigration officials.

The health impacts are injurious and enduring, as LeBrón's report indicates. "Somatic symptoms of stress responses that women described included sleeplessness, headaches, anxiety, elevated blood pressure, and disordered eating. These stress response symptoms are linked with indicators of depressive symptoms and cardiovascular risk." Just as troubling, few women in this study had access to the healthcare that could mitigate these effects.

> *There is always the fear. The kids say, "Mama, police! Mama, police! Mama, police!" They are so anxious. It's distressing . . . that is where illness comes from. No one is healthy anymore, not the kids, not the adults.*
> —Alana LeBrón, quoting from a participant in a research study

Mixed-Status Families, Mental, Emotional Well-Being

Within mixed-status families, mental and emotional well-being are intimately entangled with immigration status, personal relationships, and the broader political environment.[15] Citing several of her most recent studies from the Lower Rio Grande Valley of Texas, Melo reported that while undocumented children and parents are ineligible for all publicly funded health services (except for perinatal and emergency room care), the health of U.S. citizen children is also profoundly impacted in a mixed-status family:

> *Fear of deportation and avoidance of institutions leads some mixed-status families to limit or delay services for children or withdraw from programs altogether . . . some parents opt to not enroll eligible children in [healthcare] programs with an eye toward the greater good of the family because they do*

not want to be viewed as a public charge. Some 4.5 million U.S. citizen chil-
dren with undocumented parents live in mixed-status families.[16]

Though some research suggests divisions in families with stratified access to medical resources, Melo reviewed other studies that document supportive attitudes and adaptations. For instance, mixed-status families become accustomed to sharing "leftover" medication and "counting down" medicines to see who needs it—not only within the family but in the wider community. Despite obvious problems caused by saving doses for future uses, it is a widely known practice:[17]

> *"Aquí está la medicina que me sobró—here's the medicine that was left over." Our middle daughter always notices. When her older sister gets sick, she's the first one to say, "Mom, give her the medicine you gave me."*
> —Milena Melo, report on medicine use in mixed-status families

Being part of a mixed-status family affects the mental health and well-being of all its members. "While possessing U.S. citizenship may remove certain stressors for some, they may still be affected by worry about their loved one's undocumented or precarious status," according to a study by Melo and her colleagues.[18] Again, a host of physical symptoms often reflected their fear and anxiety.

Melo acknowledged that some immigration communities buy into the rhetoric of the "good" versus "bad" immigrant, and whether someone "came the right way" or "came the legal way." "We see this constantly trickle into the health system, where we have lots of foreign doctors who come in and judge the undocumented immigrants," said Melo. The message they are sending, she acknowledged sadly, is, "Go back to Mexico! That's your only solution. We can't treat you here."

Detention, Separation, Health Harms to Children

The detention of immigrant children and separation from family members pose long-term negative health and development threats to children. Separating parents and children, said LeBrón, "reminds us of the critical role that a baby's connection and stable relationship with a primary caregiver has on child socioemotional development, and teaches us about the enduring pain that detention and family separation due to deportation or hardened national boundaries can have on children. Family separation policies and practices have consequences for the current generation and for generations to come."

Key medical associations have acknowledged this impact. The American Psychological Association noted that the deportation policies carried out under past administrations could cause "serious mental health deterioration and trauma in children," and reported that separation policies harmed children.[19] And the American Academy of Pediatrics detailed the adverse effects of the detention of immigrant children and family separation on both short- and long-term health of family members.[20]

The Chilling Effect of Surveillance and ID Requirements

One question from LeBrón—"How are immigration policies affecting the health of the communities where you work?"—prompted an outpouring of emotional stories from contributors about their home communities.

Increased Border Surveillance: "You're Being Watched"

Like the majority of border residents in the Rio Grande Valley, Melo noted that she has had family on both sides of the Mexico–U.S. border for decades, if not centuries. Melo has lived in this country since she was 4 years old. Growing up undocumented, she always understood the power of surveillance to undermine health along the Texas border, where a third of the population is foreign born, a large percentage are undocumented, and over 80% speak Spanish (see Chapter 9 for more about this region). But the anecdote she shared still had the power to shock: In the 1990s, she recalled, a prominent hospital in her area "decided to outfit their security guards in green uniforms. So they would look like Border Patrol agents. To deter people from coming to the hospital."

While this practice has long stopped—and Melo is now a lawful permanent resident who plans to apply to become a U.S. citizen—her story reflects what it is like to live in a region "where you can be deported within a matter of hours. It's fear, it's anxiety, it's always there. People in other parts of the county would be detained and go into a detention center, and maybe there's time for some type of legal interview. Here? There isn't that time. Because 10 minutes and you are in Mexico."

Continuing her description, she called the border patrol "an everyday presence that makes you feel like you can't even go to the doctor. Our immigrant rights' organizations get calls, 'My daughter's really sick. Is it safe for me to go out?'" Residents have established informal communications networks, including Facebook posts and texts, to warn one another about the presence of border patrol and immigration authorities. "One of the things about being on the border is that over time, we have seen much more policing. It's hard for people like my husband—who is White and from Wyoming—to understand why I get nervous when a police officer pulls up behind me, but that's what everybody in our communities goes through on a daily basis."

Ironically, the infamous border wall is not as threatening as most would imagine, said Melo:

> For those of us who live here on the border, we treat the wall as kind of a joke, right? "That's what you are spending $7 billion a mile on?" We know it's not going to solve anything, but it did cause issues. We have this wonderful region that we call home, and it's constantly portrayed as a dangerous place, a place that needs to be highly surveilled, a place that needs to always be under a watchful eye because we have all of these, quote, 'illegals,' so it must be the most dangerous place.
>
> We've had the Border Patrol, traffic checkpoints, the Wall, and now we have these big blimps in the sky. And they are a visual representation of what we feel all the time: "You're being watched."

—Milena Melo

Away from the Border, But Still Terrified

In Cicero, Illinois, a suburb of Chicago where 45% of residents identify as immigrants, the fear associated with deportation and surveillance was so great that Mariana Osoria of Cicero Community Collaborative and the outreach organization Family Focus began to see a trend she had never seen in such high numbers: Families were unenrolling from programs that had nothing to do with immigration and everything to do with their family's health.

"I'm worried. I'm afraid. I don't want to be part of the program anymore." Osoria hears that from individuals who are so terrified of being deported that they drop out of essential programs like home health visits that monitor immunizations, provide well-baby visits, connect families to primary care doctors, and provide family support services. "So what we've seen in our community is increased levels of depression, of stress, anxiety, concern—immigrant families continuing to be afraid to participate in programs even if they are not impacted by the rules or proposed changes."

Osoria recalled the story of a Latino father, a legal, permanent U.S. resident who was detained by Immigration and Customs Enforcement (ICE) for several weeks. While he had diabetes, he was not given medication or permitted to see a doctor while he was detained. "This had a profound impact on his family and they will not access services. That illustrates what we've been seeing in terms of how an immigration policy impacts not just the individual but whole families."

Health Equity in a Water Bottle

Another trend with a disproportionate impact on immigrant populations is the requirement for identity cards issued by the federal, state, or local authorities. These include driver's licenses, passports, and other official IDs, which most documented individuals take for granted but that are largely unattainable for undocumented people.

LeBrón has studied how restrictive identification policies and the increasing demand for photo IDs impact health equity—documentation can be required to enter a federal building, open a bank account, get medical care, receive food stamps, or even purchase food in a grocery store. The right documents can also be the only way people can protect themselves in interactions with law enforcement agencies.[21] LeBrón described the outrageous insistence that residents of Flint, Mich., have an ID to access publicly distributed bottled water after the city's water supply had been poisoned.[22] This example, she noted, illustrated the "increasingly critical link between photo identification issued by U.S. governmental entities and access to health-promoting resources." Calling restrictive ID policies a "public health call to action," LeBrón argued that "because IDs now serve as gateways to health-promoting resources, ID policy is health policy This points to the need to address state ID policies to be more inclusive."[23]

Towards that goal, 16 states and the District of Columbia have enacted laws to allow undocumented individuals to obtain driver's licenses with a foreign birth certificate, foreign passport, or evidence of current residency in the state.[24] Despite this progress, the strengthened effort to enforce the REAL ID Act of 2005 is a looming threat to immigrant communities. This federal law, passed by Congress after the events of September 11, 2001, established specific minimum federal standards for identity cards and is scheduled to take effect on May 3, 2023. REAL ID, said LeBrón, "will strengthen a national pattern of state-issued driver's licenses and state IDs serving as markers of legal status . . . The government-issued ID climate is indeed getting worse. It is imperative that we strengthen our resolve to advocate for policies that will promote social and health equity and identify strategies to disrupt the linkages between restrictive ID policies and health."

The Impact of COVID-19

When the COVID-19 pandemic struck in the winter of 2020, the disparate impact became apparent almost immediately. Although not every geographical area reports COVID-19 case data by race and ethnicity, the Centers for Disease Control and Prevention (CDC) found that "racial and ethnic minority groups are disproportionately represented among COVID-19 cases."[25] The CDC also reported a noticeably higher percentage of COVID-19 cases among Hispanic or Latino people, especially adults under 50 and children younger than 18. Data gaps make it difficult to tease out the number of immigrants within each population group, but the harm to their communities has been clear.

In addition to infection levels, deaths from COVID-19 are far higher among racial and ethnic minority groups compared to the percentage of the total U.S. population they represent.[26] Specifically, the death rate from COVID-19 in Black, Latino, and tribal communities is at least double that of Whites and even higher among Latino populations ages 35 to 49.[27] In California, Native Hawaiians and Pacific Islanders are three times more likely to contract the disease compared to Whites, and nearly twice as likely to die. Sixteen states track their COVID death rates separately from other Asian Americans and in 11 of those states, they are dying at the highest rates of any racial or ethnic group.[28]

The numbers of excess deaths from all causes (that is, deaths beyond what would be expected in a typical year) also skews against non-White populations, sparking what has been called a "hidden crisis."[29] In the first six months of 2020, the CDC reported that excess deaths increased 14.7% for White people, 44.9% for Latinos, and 28.1% among Black populations. The result was a drop in life expectancy in the United States by a full year, on average, in the general population and by about three years among Latinos.[30]

> We're definitely living through something unique. I've never seen a disease or a virus that so discriminates against those who are the most vulnerable.
>
> —Milena Melo

Beyond its health impact, the COVID-19 pandemic has had a profoundly uneven impact on financial security. By April 2020, nearly six in 10 non-elderly Latino adults were in families where someone had lost a job, work hours, or work-related income, according to an RWJF-funded study by Urban Institute researchers.[31] The study found that Hispanic adults in families with noncitizens disproportionately work in industries that are more likely to be affected by the pandemic and experience higher levels of unemployment. These families had to cut back on spending for food (more than half worried about having enough to eat in the next month); postpone crucial household purchases; cut into savings or increase credit card debt; and worry about being able to pay electric bills, rent or mortgage, and medical costs.

LeBrón agreed that mixed-status communities and families with noncitizens have been hit particularly hard. "Mixed-status communities have shared concerns about the impact of getting COVID-19 on the health and the well-being of their families, but also on the security of their fragile jobs, housing, and immigration records," LeBrón said. Those concerns have also influenced the decision to sign up for vaccines, given fears that it could fall under the public charge rule and undermine their hopes for a path to legalization.

Seen through the lens of this country's immigration crisis, COVID-19 comes into clear focus for yet another group: tens of thousands of adults and children fighting deportation and held in more than 200 immigration centers. According to a recent article in the *American Journal of Public Health*,[32] adults and children are uniquely vulnerable to coronavirus outbreaks in these detention centers, where "infection and death from a novel communicable disease will deepen inequities for a population group that already experiences many structural and systemic threats to health and well-being." Despite compelling evidence of increased risk, the study found that "state and federal governments have done little to protect the health of detained immigrants." Though the Biden administration announced in March 2021 that it wanted every adult in the United States eligible for vaccination by May, ICE's network of jails holding civil immigration detainees had no vaccination program and could not say how many detainees had been vaccinated.[33]

> *In minority communities, we see SO many matters of life and death—immigrant policing, police violence, White supremacy, structural racism, and now COVID-19. We have a long road ahead.*
>
> —Alana LeBrón

Pursuing Positive Change

Despite LeBrón's recognition of the long road ahead, each contributor presented snapshots of success and hope in battling systems that discriminate against immigrants.

Harris County, Tex., opened a dialysis center to serve uninsured people, a category that includes many undocumented individuals. One in three people in the border region where Milena Melo works has diabetes and more than 30% of them don't know it. Fearful of seeking medical attention, they often go undiagnosed and untreated, which too often leads to kidney failure. Life-saving dialysis can cost thousands of dollars for a single treatment; the three-times-a-week dialysis routine that is the standard of care is unavailable to people who are undocumented and lack access to public insurance. After the first dialysis center to serve the uninsured opened in Harris County, the demand was so great that county officials soon expanded its hours to run dialysis machines around the clock.

Eventually, the county also opened another center, began to conduct diabetes screenings at local food markets, and connected people to a federally qualified health center, all without asking questions about immigration status.

Cities like Albuquerque, N.M., Chelsea and Revere, Mass., and Cicero, Ill., chose to take the health and safety of immigrants into their own hands. In May 2019, the Albuquerque City Council voted to spend $250,000 to help care for the 2,000 asylum seekers who had been brought to the city by the Department of Homeland Security since March.[34] "This should not be a political issue," noted one city resident who supported the expenditure. "This is a human issue. Please, be human."

In the spring of 2020, a COVID-19 surge hit Chelsea, a community with a large population of immigrants, more than 60% of them Latino and some of them undocumented. Healthcare leaders in this *RWJF Culture of Health Prize*–winning community and in nearby Revere turned a local hotel into a safe, free isolation facility for infected people who could not socially distance at home and had little access to healthcare. The hotel stayed open until early June, when the city's surge in infections subsided.[35]

In Cicero—another *RWJF Culture of Health Prize*–winning community that is a Latino-majority town, where 45% of all residents identify as immigrants—community leaders like Osoria are working to combat crime and gang violence by empowering residents of all ages.[36] Through the Cicero Community Collaborative, they have rallied to keep their school-based health clinic open, prevent violence on school routes, provide safe and enriching after-school programming, and increase access to early education (see the Spotlight at the end of this chapter).

Municipalities committed to supporting immigrants are helping to ensure that law enforcement respects their rights. Mark Hall said these steps include a "cite-and-release" approach to minor offenses to avoid an automatic query to ICE; separating law enforcement involvement from social services; discontinuing or avoiding 287(g) agreements; and reducing occasions when officers inquire about immigration status. When municipalities reduced their participation in federal immigration enforcement initiatives, immigrants reported that they "have a chance to breathe," said Hall. "Immigrants felt safer leaving their homes to meet basic needs because they felt more confident that, if stopped by local law enforcement, they would not face detention or deportation."

A Final Word

A flurry of executive orders in the early months of 2021 began to lift some of the restrictions that had been imposed on immigrant populations over the previous four years. Among other steps, the new administration in Washington moved quickly to reopen the country to people seeking green cards, noting that it was "not detrimental to the interests of the United States;" restored DACA; increased the number of refugees who can be settled here; declared a 100-day moratorium on deportations; initiated efforts to reunite children separated from their families; took steps to process claims of asylum seekers at the Mexican border; and proposed an eight-year path to citizenship for most of the 10.5 million undocumented immigrants living in the United States.[37]

Throughout this period, RWJF made its own efforts to address structural racism related to immigration, as showcased by these examples:

- In late 2020 and 2021, the Foundation supported the work of the American Civil Liberties Union Foundation to reunify and support separated immigrant families and to recalibrate U.S. immigration policy to protect asylum seekers. RWJF also provided support to the National Immigration Law Center's efforts to advance humane and inclusive immigration policies designed to enhance well-being and safety and end family separations.[38]
- In a series of policy briefs issued in January 2021, RWJF addressed inequities in housing, food, and health insurance access for immigrant communities and flagged federal policies that have the effect of discriminating based on race. Included were recommendations to "help people through the immediate health and economic crisis to ensure that all people in the United States have a fair and just opportunity to be as healthy as possible."[39]
- To help data researchers understand the extent of pandemic-related health disparities among Native Hawaiians and Pacific Islanders, RWJF awarded a grant to the Fielding School of Public Health at the University of California, Los Angeles (UCLA) to support a groundbreaking study on the impact of COVID-19 on that population.[40] "It's vital that public health data researchers in the U.S. change how we collect race and ethnicity information in population health surveys," said Ninez A. Ponce, PhD, director of Fielding's Center for Health Policy Research. "To understand vast differences between the Asian and NHPI [Native Hawaiian and Pacific Islander] experiences, we cannot keep lumping them together. If we don't make this change, we'll never achieve health equity."[41] (For more on opportunities to reimagine research and evaluation centered on equity, see Chapter 10).

Despite what they each saw as progress, all of the contributors to this chapter remained cautious about the challenges ahead. As the current administration wrestled with how to care for an estimated 35,000 unaccompanied minors who had joined the waves of people crossing the border by April 2021,[42] both Osoria and Melo stressed that health problems will escalate unless sounder immigration, health, and mental health policies are adopted. Melo and LeBrón believe that creating a pathway to citizenship for parents and siblings is the most basic step to improving the health and well-being of all immigrant children, citizens and noncitizens alike.[43] LeBrón also emphasized the urgency of disinvesting in and abolishing immigrant detention centers and investing in community-based institutions to support immigrant communities.

LeBrón thinks it will take generations to undo the effects of recent immigration policies and practices, along with the narrative of White supremacy that it amplified. "True repair," she said, "will involve undoing each of these policies and creating policies that are more inclusive of immigrants. In addition to tackling structural racism, it will take time to shift the cultural aspects of racism that have increased in the early 21st century."

And Hall warned that the physical and mental health problems now apparent in immigrant populations will not soon disappear: "These problems are getting embedded generationally. These are not problems that run their course. Once they dig in roots, they are hard to dig out."

Spotlight

Creative Approaches to Support Immigrant Families

Mariana Osoria, MA, Senior Vice President, Partnerships &
Engagement, Family Focus

Residents of Cicero, Ill.—a Latino-majority suburb of Chicago where 45% of residents identify as immigrants—have for years taken steps to improve community health outcomes as they fought back against the crime and gang violence that once threatened their community.

A recipient of the 2018 RWJF Culture of Health Prize, Cicero highlighted efforts by community members and organizations to make school settings safer and to provide mental health counseling and trainings to foster awareness of the negative effects of trauma and combat its impact.

Similar on-the-ground efforts characterize the creative approaches Cicero has embraced to address inequity and support immigrant families during a particularly threatening time for their communities, according to Mariana Osoria of Family Focus. Recently merged with Chicago Child Care Society, Family Focus offers services to families in early childhood development, youth development, and family support that help caregivers gain skills and confidence.

"Imagine not knowing the language, having to learn a new community and the structure of a city, sometimes not knowing anyone else," she said. "Navigating services can be really challenging."

> *We want to make sure that everyone in the town of Cicero feels welcome . . .*
> *this is their community.*
>
> —Mariana Osoria

Mariana Osoria, *Spotlight* In: *Necessary Conversations.* Edited by: Alonzo L. Plough, Oxford University Press. © Robert Wood Johnson Foundation 2022. DOI: 10.1093/oso/9780197641477.003.0010

Cicero Community Collaborative and Illinois Welcoming Center

Osoria described two local approaches that are designed to support immigrant families in Cicero.

Cicero Community Collaborative (CCC)

Formerly the Cicero Youth Task Force, which focused on disconnected youth, this collaborative program joins multiple sectors and residents to provide a continuum of care to young people, helping them learn to navigate nearly every system they might encounter—from health, mental health, and immigration services to early childhood programs and schooling from K to 12.

As it evolved, CCC began to engage parents, developing an expanded parent and youth ambassador program that Osoria said "changed the conversation... It had more people talking about issues from many different perspectives, and thinking about both prevention and intervention." As part of a visioning session, youth and their parents came together to ask, "What do we want in the town of Cicero? What are the gifts and strengths that people already bring?" No one was ever asked to show an identity document to participate in these conversations, and the answers that emerged helped CCC refine its vision and continue to grow.

The ambassador program is just one example of a support network that has expanded in Cicero through CCC to help immigrants know their rights and connect with services. Osoria and Family Focus also work through CCC to provide employment strategies to help individuals secure and keep jobs; support for everything from finding places to live to signing up for utilities; and guidance on navigating the health system, including disseminating information about COVID-19. Still another activity is rapid response training to prepare immigration advocates to respond when a community faces a raid by ICE personnel. At the scene, they document what is happening and disseminate information to support the impacted family or individual.

All told, CCC has developed a platform to bring people together to define local needs, agree on priorities, and take actions that give everyone a chance at a healthier life. It is also helping to create a new generation of leaders who have lived the immigrant experience themselves.

Illinois Welcoming Center

Osoria noted that Illinois is intentionally a welcoming state to immigrants; since 1975, almost 124,000 refugees from more than 60 countries have settled there.[1] The Welcoming Center model places comprehensive service centers run by nonprofit organizations, including Family Focus, in communities with a high percentage of immigrants and refugees to help settle families into their new lives. Each center connects families with important state and local services, ranging from healthcare and food pantries to immigration experts and housing, eliminating systemic barriers that immigrants may otherwise face.[2] "It's a one-stop-shop, because it certainly can connect that family to the right services," said Osoria. "I always like to say, 'It is the expert on the experts.'"

Osoria noted that many other programs supportive of immigrants are now embedded in Family Focus, CCC, and Welcoming Center sites, engaging local school boards, nonprofit organizations, and government agencies. As these organizations tackle issues of racism and discrimination, Osoria seeks change in every corner, including police and healthcare. She argued that while Cook County Health and Hospital Systems provides the level of charity care required of nonprofit systems, other large hospital systems and teaching institutions in the Chicago–Cicero area do not. "They are not doing their fair share," she said, noting that the Illinois Coalition for Immigrant and Refugee Rights has embraced health as one of its core issues and will be working to improve access to services.

Osoria recognizes that the pandemic and the immigration crisis in this country have escalated substance use and mental health issues, something that Family Focus and CCC work continuously address. Osoria is especially concerned about young people. "Because of that fear and trauma and heightened anxiety, I'm very concerned about what young adolescents and young children will be facing as we move forward. It's going to be very challenging," she said. "But I feel incredibly fortunate to be able to work in Cicero, one of the few collaborative community areas that has really been able to see efforts across sectors that have broad impact."

Climate Crisis, Environmental Justice, and Racial Justice

Robert D. Bullard, PhD, Distinguished Professor of Urban Planning and Environmental Policy and Director of Bullard Center for Environmental and Climate Justice Barbara Jordan-Mickey Leland School of Public Affairs, Texas Southern University

Ronda Lee Chapman, Director of Equity, The Trust for Public Land; former Senior Associate, PolicyLink

Chris M. Kabel, Senior Fellow, The Kresge Foundation

Nyiesha Mallett, Climate Justice Youth Organizer, UPROSE

Jackie Qataliña Schaeffer, Senior Project Manager, Alaska Native Tribal Health Consortium

For more than 40 years, the environmental justice movement has focused on the intersectionality of climate change, environmental hazards, racism, and health—building from landmark litigation in 1979 documenting that nearly all of the waste dumped in Houston was concentrated in Black neighborhoods.[1,2]

But not everyone paid attention. Certainly, not everyone acted after the first clear-cut case of environmental racism went to court. Though efforts to make the environmental justice movement a unifying theme across race, class, gender, and geographical lines persisted for decades, the inequities nationwide remained stark. By 2020, people of color in almost every state lived with more air and chemical pollution than Whites; lacking green space, poor neighborhoods were far hotter than wealthier ones; and communities that are economically vulnerable, as well as communities that are majority non-White, continued to bear the brunt of climate change and its health-damaging effects.[3]

Robert D. Bullard, Ronda Lee Chapman, Chris M. Kabel, Nyiesha Mallett, and Jackie Qataliña Schaeffer, *Climate Crisis, Environmental Justice, and Racial Justice* In: *Necessary Conversations.* Edited by: Alonzo L. Plough, Oxford University Press. © Robert Wood Johnson Foundation 2022. DOI: 10.1093/oso/9780197641477.003.0011

The consequences of climate change, the devastating coronavirus pandemic, and the explosion of racial protests finally pushed environmental justice to the forefront. In 2020, the very wording of the conversation shifted to reflect new urgency. The term climate "change" evolved to climate "crisis" as the world experienced the highest temperature on record.[4] Experts began to replace the phrase "natural disasters" with "climate disasters," which more adequately described the unprecedented number of catastrophic fires, hurricanes, and flooding that year.[5]

Also in 2020, the World Health Organization identified health and climate as the number-one global health priority. Moreover, spurred by the reckoning with the racial inequity that was underscored by the pandemic, police brutality, and economic injustice, the term "environmental racism" gained footing to describe the disproportionate risks of the combined crises in communities of color.[6]

This chapter begins with author and scholar Robert D. Bullard, justifiably called the "father of environmental justice," who reviews the health impacts of the climate crisis and how the pandemic and racial injustice uprisings combined to push the movement forward. Next, Ronda Chapman focuses on water equity and its troubling ties to climate injustice and COVID-19. Jackie Qataliña Schaeffer of the Alaska Native Tribal Health Consortium (ANTHC) describes the unique water challenges her community faces with climate change at its front door.

Chris Kabel of The Kresge Foundation and RWJF's Alonzo Plough then look through the lens of inequity to review the partnerships their foundations have embraced to advance environmental justice, while 20-year-old Nyiesha Mallett celebrates the importance of youth in the movement. The chapter ends on a distinct message of hope, born from action taken swiftly by a new administration in 2021 that has prioritized environmental justice for the first time in a generation.

Dumping on People of Color—Literally

Robert Bullard traces his introduction to the environmental justice movement back to 1979, when as a sociology professor at Texas Southern University he worked with several of his research students to document how the overwhelming preponderance of landfill waste dumped in Houston from the 1930s until 1979 went to Black neighborhoods.[7]

More specifically, Bullard's wife, attorney Linda McKeever Bullard, had asked him to conduct a study in support of the *Bean v. Southwestern Waste Management Corp.* lawsuit she had filed against the City of Houston, Harris County, the state of Texas, and Browning Ferris Industries, the second-largest waste disposal company in the country, headquartered in Houston. Working with students in his research methods class, Bullard showed that over 82% of the solid waste dumped in Houston over five decades went to Black neighborhoods, even though Black Houstonians represented approximately 25% of the city's total population.

Bullard soon discovered that what was happening in Houston was mirrored across the South, and it was not an accident. "Systemic racism created these unequal, invisible communities that receive the worst of the worst," he argued. In 1990, he published *Dumping in Dixie: Race, Class, and Environmental Quality*, perhaps the first book to explore environmental racism and environmental justice in depth. Since then, Bullard's extensive studies of regions hardest hit by flooding, high temperatures, and other markers of climate change have shown how closely they overlap with regions plagued by inequities in health outcomes, income, education, and housing, and that those inequities invariably fall along racial and ethnic lines.

> *Is climate change fair? I can answer that in two words: "Hell no."*
> —Robert Bullard

The Climate Crisis Consequences That Other People Don't Want

For over 40 years and in 18 books, Bullard has delivered one basic message: "Communities of color and low-income communities get more than their fair share of things that other people don't want."

Bullard's list of "things that other people don't want" includes:

- **Air pollution.** In 46 states, people of color live with more air pollution than White people. Black people are exposed to 1.54 times more fine particulate matter than White people; Latinos 1.2 times; and those living below poverty 1.35 times more than those living above poverty.[8]
- **Flooding and an inadequate government response after a disaster**. A recent study of Hurricane Harvey found that storm-induced flooding was significantly greater in Houston neighborhoods with a higher proportion of Black and poor residents. The same trends have been reported following devastating storms and storm surges in New Orleans and Charleston, S.C.[9] Strong and consistent evidence demonstrates that government response to natural and human-made disasters over the past eight decades has not treated all communities equally, a lesson that people of color along the Gulf Coast witnessed dramatically after the delayed response to Hurricane Katrina jeopardized their lives.[10]
- **Extreme heat.** Described as "one of the most important manifestations of climate change on health," study after study has found that heat-related deaths

among Black people occur at a 150% to 200% greater rate than for White people; that low-income neighborhoods are hotter than wealthier ones; and that extreme heat caused by climate change has disproportionately impacted historically underserved populations and vulnerable communities, particularly those living in "heat islands" characterized by an abundance of concrete and pavements and lack of green spaces and tree canopies.[11]

- **Illness and disease.** In 2019, Black children were five times more likely than White children to be hospitalized for asthma and eight times more likely to die from the condition, which can be triggered or worsened by pollution.[12] Children, older adults, people with low incomes, and communities of color disproportionately bear the burden of climate change–related illnesses, including respiratory illnesses like asthma, heat-related illnesses, and diseases spread by ticks and mosquitos.[13]

- **Economic and income disparity, with poor people and people of color in the South hit hardest.** Bullard argues that environmental disasters widen racial wealth gaps. Citing research on disasters that caused at least $10 billion in damage in communities, Bullard noted that White households gain an average of $126,000 in personal wealth while households of color average losses of up to $29,000.[14] The government response is a contributing factor, said Bullard: "The money that gets sent down to places generally goes to rich White communities that can recover quickly. Communities of color generally lose."

Environmental racism kills. It makes people sick. The environmental justice movement grew out of the fight for civil rights and human rights, but when we bring them all together, it's just one movement: the movement for justice.
—Robert Bullard

The Intersection of Climate Change, Structural Racism, and COVID-19

Just before Bullard's presentation in Jackson, RWJF's Alonzo Plough asked the question: "Why hasn't the impact of climate on health and well-being gotten more deeply into the minds of folks? You know, *what does it take?*" That was the first week of March 2020. The country would soon realize that COVID-19 was disproportionately sickening people of color, landing them in hospitals with lung and respiratory ailments, and sometimes killing them. *"I can't breathe."* Within months of COVID's swift emergence, the George Floyd murder in Minneapolis would prove to be a tipping point, sparking an outcry against long-standing racial inequities and police brutality that to this day has not been silenced. *"I can't breathe."* In many ways, Plough got his answer: It took a global pandemic and a national uprising against racism to finally align climate change and health.

Not long after the first traces of the pandemic emerged, experts drew the parallels. To wit: Like climate change, the virus that causes COVID-19 puts everyone at risk, but people of color face the most dire consequences. As former Secretary of State and climate crisis czar John Kerry wrote, "The parallels between COVID-19 and climate change are screaming at us." And similar to climate change and COVID-19, the criminal justice system disproportionately targets Black people, who are more likely than White people to be stopped by the police[15] and who greatly outnumber Whites in the country's prisons.[16] This undeniable spotlight on health and racial inequities in a multiplicity of venues gave visibility to what environmental justice advocates like Bullard have been saying for decades.

"What's different with this is that we have the video of Black men and women being shot, killed, choked, playing over and over and over," Bullard concluded. "And with everything about climate and health—the elevated asthma, respiratory disease, strokes, diabetes—we've got the statistics but we don't have the video of the Black kids dying from asthma at 10 times the rate of White kids. Those statistics are invisible. Yes, they're in the journals and the articles, but they don't make the headlines and the six o'clock news. But these televised lynchings of Black men and women? That hit a nerve unlike any nerve that's been hit. It's out now. And no, it's not going back."

> Black people have been saying "we can't breathe" for decades. It just took this long for everyone to hear us.[17]
>
> —Robert Bullard

Water Equity and Climate Change Injustice

Just as it took time to fully embrace the connection between climate change and health, so too have the troubling ties between water equity and climate change injustice only been acknowledged very slowly. But that, too, is beginning to change. Two months into 2020, Jackson, Miss., had already issued three "boil water" safety alerts and experienced flooding from the nearby Pearl River, putting more pressure on a water system frequently in violation of drinking water standards and struggling with a vast network of lead pipes.[18] But few in the audience for the *Sharing Knowledge* conference knew this. "In terms of water equity, I'd like to see a show of hands of all of you who had an opportunity to have a glass of water this morning," asked conference presenter Ronda Chapman. Nearly every hand was raised. "Really fortunate, right? And it's something that we tend to take for granted."

Though the water in Jackson was safe to drink during this event, Chapman noted that Jackson residents were among some of the 77 million people in the United States—nearly one-quarter of the U.S. population—who are served by water systems that frequently violate the health-based standards established in the Safe Drinking Water Act.[19] Still others struggle to pay their water bills or are unable to access running water at all. According to the 2019 report called *Closing the Water Access Gap in the United States*:[20]

- **More than 2 million Americans live without running water and basic indoor plumbing, and many more are without sanitation.** These include the most vulnerable people in the country—low-income people in rural areas, people of color, tribal communities, immigrants, and homeless populations.
- **Native American households are 19 times more likely than White households to lack indoor plumbing.** On the Navajo Nation in the Southwest, an estimated 30% of residents do not have running water, and family members may have to drive for hours to haul barrels of water to meet their basic needs.
- **In rural areas, 17% of people report having experienced issues with safe drinking water and 12% report issues with their sewage system.** In Alabama, parents have warned their children not to play outside because their yards are flooded with sewage.

"I don't know how to answer why our water crisis is not on everyone's radar—but it's probably for the same reason that the connection between our climate crisis and its impact on health isn't either," Chapman said. "Both disproportionately impact cities and rural communities with majority Black or Indigenous populations, places where residents have been fighting for years for reliable, affordable access to safe water."[21]

While Flint, Mich., was arguably the site of one of the highest-profile public works tragedies of the past decade and a textbook case of environmental injustice,[22] it was far from unique in producing poisoned tap water. In a story Bullard called a "poster child case for toxic water racism," a Black family in Dickson County, Tenn., drank water contaminated by the chemical trichloroethylene from 1988 to 2000. White families had been warned of the contamination, but the Black family received letters assuring them that their well water was safe. In 2003, the family filed a lawsuit charging racial discrimination, ultimately settling out of court in 2011.[23]

Chapman also reminded the audience that nearly 5,000 residents near Toledo, Ohio, had been exposed to toxic drinking water from an algae bloom on

Lake Erie in 2014. "Many of the people who were impacted in Toledo were low-income and non-White residents," she said. But exemplars may sometimes mask the uniqueness of the problem, she noted: "I try not to name each situation and place because we have a crisis in so many cities and counties and small towns all across the country. It's not just one singular story."

> *Water is a human right . . . it seems counterintuitive that one of the wealth-iest nations requires so many people to fight for access to safe and affordable drinking water.*
>
> —Ronda Chapman

Water Infrastructure: Lifesaving and Economically Sound

Promoting water infrastructure to achieve water equity was Chapman's mission during her two years as senior associate at PolicyLink, a national research and action institute devoted to advancing racial and economic equity. Many key regulations governing water protection were in danger of being rolled back in the final years of the Trump administration, and newly enacted laws weakened existing standards. As a result, the mounting water crisis remains dire, as the PolicyLink website summarized:

> *Across the country, communities face mounting threats to their water secu-rity. Increased climate-change-related flooding, sea level rise, and drought threaten people's homes, lives, and the ecosystems they rely upon. Millions of Americans live in communities that do not have access to reliable safe drinking water. Many live in areas where the cost of water is unaffordable, and children across the country attend schools where their drinking water is contaminated with lead.*[24]

In April 2018, PolicyLink, with support from The Kresge Foundation, partnered with the Gulf Coast Center for Law and Policy to create the Water Equity and Climate Resilience Caucus.[25] The caucus, representing a national network of organizations working in inland, rural, and coastal communities, pledged to focus on building equity in four areas: the human right to water; access to affordable, safe drinking water and sanitation; resilience investments that address climate-related water management and equitable water systems; and educational, workforce, and business pathways to resilient water management.

Supporting an equitable, safe water infrastructure system makes economic sense, Chapman reminded the conference audience, pointing out that it represents one of the largest sectors in the U.S. economy, providing close to 300,000 utility jobs and employing another 1.5 million people in water-related activities. "Water is something that so many of us take for granted and yet we have a water crisis in the United States," said Chapman. "Our shared well-being depends on everyone having access to water."

The Interplay of Safe Water and COVID-19

The importance of Chapman's words became even more apparent as COVID-19 surged. "When you're telling folks to wash their hands and they cannot because they live in communities plagued by tainted water, crumbling sanitation systems, unaffordable water bills or service shutoffs, it gives people an opportunity to pause," said Chapman. "People have died because they didn't have access to water. In their passing, the issue is being elevated in a way that I don't think anyone was paying attention to before."

Chapman knew intuitively that the virus would immediately impact majority Black and Indigenous communities where residents had been fighting for years for reliable, affordable access to safe water. Experience proved her right: Before the pandemic, she said that an estimated 15 million people nationwide in 2020 (mostly people of color struggling with poverty and unemployment) had experienced water shutoffs for varying amounts of time when they couldn't pay their bills.[26] When COVID-19 struck, many of those same populations were hardest hit.

In Detroit, for example, "an estimated 2,800 homes were experiencing water shutoffs," wrote Chapman. Though Black Americans make up less than 14% of the Michigan population, they had accounted for nearly 40% of the coronavirus deaths by April. That pattern held in the Navajo Nation, where an estimated 30% of residents lack running water, and there are also high rates of diabetes and other health conditions that make them more vulnerable to the virus. The Navajo Nation reported almost 5,000 confirmed cases of COVID-19 by the end of May, representing one of the highest infection rates in the United States.[27]

"COVID-19 exposes the dangers and immorality of decades of underinvestment, unjust policies at all levels of government," Chapman wrote. "In essence, the policies that deprive people of color of access to drinking water are no different than any other act of unjustified violence, such as police brutality, militarized streets, and electoral injustice. We are bearing witness to the interconnected nature of it all as people are taking to the streets demanding change."[28]

> *Coronavirus has laid bare the racial fault lines in access to clean, safe water. COVID-19 is a never-ending lesson in the history, legacy, and reality of structural racism in America.*
>
> —Ronda Chapman

For Indigenous populations, water is sacred. "Indigenous communities rightly refer to water as a *relative*, reminding us that we are deeply connected to water and should treat it with respect, care, and humility," Chapman observed. "This moment of disruption creates a unique opportunity to rework our inadequate and inequitable water systems and reconceive how we value and manage them, bending the arc toward structural and just change."[29]

Indigenous Populations in Alaska

Chapman's messages on water equity, climate change, and the value of Indigenous cultures resonate deeply with Jackie Qataliña Schaeffer of the ANTHC. Born and raised north of the Arctic Circle in a centuries-old trading community called Kotzebue, Schaeffer is Inupiaq, part of the coastal and northwest Arctic Inuit tribe that has existed on Alaskan land for over 17,000 years. She was raised in a very traditional Inupiaq home, spending half the year in the community and the other half at her family's fishing camp, "living off the land, air, and sea. We were migratory people. We traveled seasonally with the food resources, living a subsistence lifestyle, collecting and gathering plants, medicinal plants and berries, hunting and fishing and preserving foods for the winter season when we lived back in Kotzebue."

No land mass, people, or habitat in Alaska is immune to climate change. The warming waters of Bering Sea, for instance, directly impact the nation's largest fisheries;[30] and the warming climate across the entire state has caused a rapid decrease in summer sea ice, shrinking glaciers, and thawing permafrost, resulting in damage to infrastructure, major changes to ecosystems, and significant threats to food security and overall well-being.[31]

All of that has changed the world that Schaeffer has known since childhood. In her community overlooking Kotzebue Sound, she charts the march of climate crisis and rising sea levels by what she sees in communities across the state, including homes perched precariously along the rising waters' edge, inhabited until they literally fall into the sea. Growing up, Schaeffer remembers Kotzebue's quarter-mile gravel beach between her home and the sea, a critical stretch for essential commerce and trade that also provided storm protection from rising sea levels. "But there is no beach now. All we have is this 20-foot sea wall, and that's been compromised twice. In my 55 years of life on this planet, I've gone from a beach to a sea wall, from being protected to being vulnerable."

We are at the frontline of climate change every day. We literally sit in the front row of nature's response to human-led actions that contribute to these changes.
—Jackie Qataliña Schaeffer

Bringing Water and Sanitation to Homes

Schaeffer readily acknowledges that her "life experience is what brought me to this work." At the ANTHC, she examines the connection between climate and health, with a focus on the lack of basic water and sanitation services. Approximately 3,300 homes in over 30 communities in rural Alaska lack in-home piped water,[32] a challenge Schaeffer knows all too well. As a child in Kotzebue, her family had no piped-in water and no septic systems. "We used ice in the winter and spring water in the summer," she said. "And we had honey buckets in our homes for sanitation."

One of seven grantees in RWJF's Health and Climate Solutions program, ANTHC is now working to assess whether a Portable Alternative Sanitation System (PASS) can improve household water security, health, and well-being in rural Alaska Native communities.[33] The individual household PASS units consist of a modular, point-of-entry water treatment and sanitation system that provides treated, gravity-fed running water, 100 gallons of water storage capacity, a separating (dry) toilet and urinal, and onsite waste disposal. All of it is designed to complement subsistence activities, reflect Indigenous knowledge and values, and be affordable. So far, nearly 90 units have been installed in climate-threatened rural communities where the changing environment has made it nearly impossible to build traditional water and sewer infrastructures.

"It costs an average of $40 million to install piped water and sewer systems in the average community in rural Alaska," explained Schaeffer. "But now the permafrost is melting, the sea ice protection is gone, and we have storm erosion and extreme storms along the coast. Which means that an entire $40 million infrastructure could be wiped away in one storm. Our communities cannot afford or sustain this traditional system, nor can investors continue to bear the cost of rebuilding."

Working Toward the Future While Respecting the Past

Schaeffer continues to investigate ways to bring water equity to Alaska's rural communities, including the possibility of using natural water resources in ways that are safe. "We're starting to shift our mindset and, like our ancestors did, we are looking at traditional water sources," she said. She constantly revisits the perspective of her ancestors, remembering stories passed from generation to generation about long stretches of hot summers or rising sea waters—natural, weather-related events never once referred to as a "crisis." Today, when she sees the Northern Lights dance, she said, "It's as though all of our ancestors are up there, reminding us, 'You have survived for 17,000 years. *Suama*—We are resilient.' Adaptability and resilience have always been in our DNA. It's important as

we face climate change and consider our well-being that we start with a foundation of resilience—not a crumbling foundation."

The challenges ahead, however, are not lost on Schaeffer: "

Our ancestors had generations to adapt to changes that we are responding to
in a single generation."

Taking on Responsibility for Environmental Justice

While environmental activists have long fought for environmental justice, the
cause is also now being championed by a broader community of leaders, ranging
from foundations to impacted communities to future generations with arguably
the most to lose.

Foundation Leadership Steps Up

RWJF's Alonzo Plough and Chris Kabel of The Kresge Foundation fully agree
that engaging and aligning the philanthropic sector to address environmental
injustice and climate crisis has never been more critical.[34] Though most health
philanthropies once saw climate action as outside their mission and stayed on
the sidelines, both RWJF and Kresge have sought in recent years to collaborate
with local, regional, and state funders to exchange ideas, develop joint strategies, and generate additional resources to address social determinants of health
through the lens of climate resilience and health equity. While their efforts as a
health foundation partnership are unique, it is not the first multiple-foundation
initiative to tackle climate change. In September 2018, nine foundations at the
Global Climate Action Summit pledged to give $429 million to support forests
and Indigenous land rights as a climate change mitigation strategy.[35]

"The urgency of climate change requires us to shed the usual siloed approaches
of institutional philanthropy and respond in a more robust and coordinated way
than ever before," noted Kabel in a statement designed to explain the collaboration between the two foundations. "We have launched connected and complementary initiatives that aim to identify and advance community-led efforts
to improve health and climate resilience, with a strong focus on health equity."
Consider:

- Through its Health and Climate Solutions initiative, RWJF is working
  with leaders in communities across the United States to identify, highlight, and learn from smart, effective approaches and solutions that improve
  health, advance health equity, and address climate change. The grantees

are contributing critical insights to explain why some people experience a greater burden of climate change harms and feel it sooner and why race, age, income, a pre-existing health condition or chronic illness, and residential and workplace location influence the harms experienced because of climate change.[36]

- The Kresge Foundation has provided grants to 15 community-based non-profit organizations and coalitions to advance equitable policy solutions aimed at improving climate resilience and reducing health risks in low-income urban communities. (One of these grantees is the advocacy organizations UPROSE, described below.) These grants were made within Kresge's Climate Change, Health and Equity initiative, which incorporates three complementary strategies: supporting community-based advocacy; building the capacity of healthcare and public health institutions to become more climate resilient; and supporting healthcare and public health practitioners to become more active in promoting climate policy solutions.[37]

"While our two approaches—building an evidence base around community efforts [RWJF], and proposing new policies and building champions [Kresge]—are different, we see them as complementary and unified," said Plough, who credits Kresge with helping RWJF design stronger pathways to address environmental inequities. "Both have a shared commitment to racial, social, and health equity. And we believe that communities experiencing the most profound effects of climate change should have the resources they need to lead climate resilience initiatives."

Leadership Centered by Those Impacted Most

Robert Bullard and others have for years emphasized that the people most impacted by environmental injustice belong at the table to discuss solutions, a process Bullard refers to as "bottom up." (For more on building community power and equity-focused participation, see the Epilogue to this book.)

"The reasons we have an environmental justice movement is because the green movement, the conservation movement, and environmental movements basically failed to address equity issues," he said, explaining why bottom-up equity leadership is so important. "The environmental movement was largely White and did not address issues of justice until we challenged that. We need to have 'justice' in the climate movement because the people who are most impacted first, worst, and longest—those front-line communities that get hit the hardest and have contributed to the problems the least—are the ones that need to have justice."

Climate change is more than "greenhouse gases" and "parts per million." It's about vulnerability, responsibility, and addressing barriers that made some people and places more vulnerable, while directing resources, policies, and actions toward making them more livable, healthy, and sustainable.

—Robert Bullard

Bullard is focused not only on shifting resources to communities impacted most by environmental injustice but also on training the next generation of leadership. To advance that commitment, he is working with environmental justice advocate Beverly Wright, PhD, executive director of the Deep South Center for Environmental Justice, to engage historically Black colleges and universities (HBCUs, as they are commonly known) in climate change initiatives.[38] To date, 35 such institutions in 19 states are participants and Bullard wants to expand that to all 104 of them. The participating colleges and universities are in states that are home to 60% of the Black population, representing some 40 million Black people. Said Bullard, "That's a lot of our people, led by the next generation of leaders."

The Next Generation of Leadership, Already at the Table

As she continues to advance the practice of intergenerational leadership, Nyiesha Mallett, age 20, believes she also reflects the historical role of Black and Brown youth in the struggle for environmental justice:

Our voice is super important because we are the ones who are most affected by the climate crisis. We're just continuing the conversation that our ancestors started when they were young. It's the cycle of life for me.

Now in her second year at Cooper Union, which offers undergraduate and graduate degree programs in New York City's East Village, Mallett is an aspiring artist. She started working with UPROSE when she was 14, landing a summer internship with this Brooklyn-based, grassroots organization that prides itself on being intergenerational, multiracial, and led by women of color to promote sustainability and resiliency. Mallett never left.

As a climate justice youth organizer for UPROSE, she has worked alongside others to shut down power plants, create green space, and fight displacement and gentrification in the Brooklyn neighborhood of Sunset Park. Seeing every opportunity as a responsibility, Mallett also helped to assemble the largest-ever U.S. gathering of young people of color for the Climate Justice Youth Summit and represented UPROSE at the United Nations Climate Change Conference and the Conference of the Parties (COP25) in December 2019.

"From the Black Panthers, Young Lords, Purpose Berets, and American Indian movements, young people of color have always been at the forefront of fighting for justice," she said. "Climate change and the history of extraction—which created generational health disparities and increased our vulnerabilities to the impacts of climate injustice—are not different. Young people have been fighting to help move our communities away from the extraction economy to one that honors our people and our Mother Earth. The work that we do at UPROSE is at the intersection of climate justice and racial justice. We are happy when that conversation is being had. And in 2020, I think climate justice was one of the top conversations."

Mallett said that while she has not personally experienced any discrimination within the movement, she does see "a lot of helicoptering into communities of color. What I mean by 'helicopter' is that White-led, Big Greens move into communities of color to address climate change when local grassroots community organizations are already doing the work. They come not knowing anything about the community trying to implement their own solutions."

Like Bullard, she believes that the solutions should come from "on-the-ground folks who are most impacted by the issues. It should be the frontline communities impacted the most developing and implementing the solutions, connecting to that Indigenous way of thinking of protecting the land that we are living on."

Despite considerable efforts, Mallett said the past four years have made it challenging to build leadership within communities of color "when my peers are faced with racial violence, deportation threats, police harassment, and other challenges." And yet she is very hopeful: "Once they understand how these topics are interconnected, they will understand the importance of their voice in the movement."

A Final Word

In January 2021, a moment four decades in the making finally became a reality: The words of an entire environmental justice movement had not only been *heard* but were being *embraced* in Washington, D.C. Quite literally, the language of this 40-year-old movement was suddenly being spoken and incorporated into presidential acts, congressional resolutions, proposed legislation, and stimulus package proposals designed to acknowledge and address long-standing inequities. The idioms of racial and health inequity, environmental justice, water inequities, and climate crisis suddenly became commonplace.

By the end of January 2021, newspapers had reported that the new administration had promised to make "tackling America's persistent racial and economic disparities" a central part of a plan "to combat climate change, prioritizing environmental justice for the first time in a generation."[39] Officials moved quickly to establish a White House Interagency Council on Environmental Justice; rejoined the Paris Climate Accord that seeks to limit global warming; directed the Department of Health and Human Services to establish an Office of Climate Change and Health Equity; and formed a separate environmental justice office at the U.S. Justice Department to expand the department's existing work.

In addition, agencies across the federal government were directed to invest in low-income and minority communities that have traditionally borne the brunt of pollution, with an order for the government to spend 40% of its sustainability investments on disadvantaged communities.[40] And when the COVID-19 stimulus package was announced in early March 2021, it included $100 million in funding for action on air pollution and environmental health risks in marginalized communities.[41]

For Bullard and so many others involved for so long in the movement, it was the ultimate confirmation that voices for environmental justice had finally been heard. "The converging environmental, economic, and health threats from COVID-19, the racial justice awakening, and the 2020 national election outcome had clearly moved environmental justice from a footnote to a headline," he said. The 2020 recipient of the United Nations' "Champions of the Earth Lifetime Achievement Award," Bullard recognized that his life's work was now fully embraced.[42]

When you have the most powerful legal department in the country saying that environmental justice is a basic right, I think that is a signal being sent across the country. This is real, at the highest level.

—Robert Bullard

PART III

STRATEGIES TO ADVANCE RACIAL EQUITY

Acknowledging the framework that bolsters institutional racism, as outlined in Part I, and its impact on specific populations, as explored in Part II, contributors to this section consider opportunities to use societal structures and systems to move toward greater health and racial equity. Strategies emerge by paying attention to history, place, the development and use of knowledge, and the civic engagement that gives people a voice in guiding the country forward. Together these can diminish the reach of racist influences and foster racial equity in health and healthcare by changing narratives, attitudes, policies, and practices.

Chapter 8, "Learning the Lessons of History," dives into the present-day impact of the centuries in which Black people have been maltreated—from the brutality of slavery to the failure to support neighborhood opportunity to violence at the hands of the police. In probing this history—about which many people, especially White people, are unaware—three researchers also describe the benefits of educating everyone about it. A fourth researcher describes a community-wide effort to investigate the health effects of preserving civil rights sites, events, and memories.

Local environments are a major influence on health and well-being, and discriminatory housing practices allow structural racism to undermine health equity. Chapter 9, "Fair Housing, Equitable Communities," showcases the power of strengthening communities and increasing access to affordable, quality housing in neighborhoods of opportunity. Building on findings from the Child Opportunity Index that document significant disparities across neighborhoods, contributors discuss the risks and benefits of zoning and land use reforms, ways to ensure meaningful housing choice, and tactics for helping very low-income people build home equity.

Traditional research and evaluation frameworks and methodologies have been anchored in the values and perspectives of the White-dominant culture, with often scant attention paid to those of Black, Latino, Indigenous, Asian American, and other populations of color. The contributors to Chapter 10, "Transforming Research and Evaluation," offer new ways of thinking about these practices through the lens of racial equity, inclusion, and social justice, employing the full range of methods through which people share knowledge. This broader view helps to identify and guide equitable policies and strategies directed at health and well-being.

The section closes by considering two essential elements of civic society in Chapter 11, "Racial Justice Through Civic Engagement: A Look at Voting and the Census." A stable, thriving democracy committed to racial equity and justice requires that many voices be included in the public discourse. Voting gives individuals a say in the direction of their communities, regions, and country while census participation ensures that institutions reflect all of those who live in the United States and that communities receive their fair share of public goods and services. Three contributors reflect on the promise and reality of engaging with the voting process and the census, and on the divisive political climate that threatens both of these foundations of democracy.

Learning the Lessons of History

Madeline England, MIA, Former Community Health Director, Mississippi State Department of Health

Cristy Johnston Limón, MBA, Former Executive Director, Youth Speaks

Byron D'Andra Orey, PhD, Professor of Political Science, Jackson State University

Jason Reece, PhD, Assistant Professor, City and Regional Planning, Ohio State University

Geoff K. Ward, PhD, Professor of African and African-American Studies, Washington University in St. Louis

The ways in which history is remembered, analyzed, memorialized, and taught can help heal divisions among groups through shared understanding, or it can lead to continued injustice and exacerbate inequity. As it confronts the history of racist violence and discrimination in the United States, this chapter offers perspectives on its enduring impact and suggests ways to use history as a framework to promote justice and health equity.

The intertwined legacies of government- and community-sanctioned violence and discrimination against Black people are evident in the health, social, and economic status of Black people today. Three researchers address the contemporary impact of centuries of history on the day-to-day life experiences and physical and emotional health of Black individuals, families, and communities, and offer ways forward.[1] Historical sociologist Geoff K. Ward from Washington University in St. Louis connects the brutal history of lynching and slavery to current levels of violence, while also emphasizing the restorative potential of "memory work." Ohio State University city and regional planning researcher

Madeline England, Cristy Johnston Limón, Byron D'Andra Orey, Jason Reece, and Geoff K. Ward, *Learning the Lessons of History* In: *Necessary Conversations*. Edited by: Alonzo L. Plough, Oxford University Press. © Robert Wood Johnson Foundation 2022. DOI: 10.1093/oso/9780197641477.003.0012

Jason Reece acknowledges the role of past housing policies in shaping the opportunities available for the Black population today and explains the value of teaching that history. Political scientist Byron D'Andra Orey at Jackson State University explores the physiological and emotional impacts of racist symbols and how understanding those impacts can drive change.

In an example from the field, Madeline England, former community health researcher at the Mississippi State Department of Health, shares insights about the health impact of addressing civil rights historical preservation in a Mississippi River community. Finally, in the Spotlight at the end of the chapter, former Youth Speaks executive director Cristy Johnston Limón advocates for youth taking charge of the historical narratives thrust upon them and raising their voices for change.

Lifting the "Veil of Oblivion"

When studying the racial history of juvenile justice, Geoff K. Ward, professor of African and African-American studies at Washington University, became very interested in what he called "the historical arc of racial violence." Black leaders, especially Black women—"Black child savers," in his words—fought against a system of juvenile justice that had been organized to privilege White youth and disadvantage non-White youth. The Black child savers framed this Jim Crow form of justice as a "genocidal institution that was 'killing the seeds of a people,'" said Ward. They understood it for what it was—a tool that cemented collective economic, social, political, and health inequality.[2]

Ward's interest in this legacy led to research that showed a strong correlation between histories of racial violence and current-day patterns of conflict, violence, and inequity. He wanted to understand how the trauma of slavery, lynching, and other systematic violence becomes embedded in the social fabric of today—and what can be done to counter these effects. (While Ward's work focuses on historical connections with the contemporary experiences of Black people, he emphasized that the present-day dynamics resulting from a history of racial violence have implications for all members of a racialized social system and that the promotion of justice and health equity has wide-ranging benefits, including for the dominant group.[3])

Acknowledgment and Memory

After a Black man was burned to death in a brutal lynching in St. Louis, Mo., in 1836, the editors of the *Missouri Republican* recommended that "the veil of oblivion be drawn over the fatal affair," as if it had never happened.[4] Ward argued, "We've been doing that for some time, but it doesn't make the history irrelevant to the organization of our society. It's still there; it's just unacknowledged and unaddressed."

Lynching is the most fully documented and most extensively studied form of racial violence. The number of lynchings in a county or cluster of counties has been shown to predict a range of contemporary outcomes, including the number of homicides in which Black people are the victims.[5] But community characteristics can influence the strength of this association. Ward cited a 2017 study that explored local "indicators of resistance" to continuing this legacy.[6] In particular, researchers found a weaker link between lynchings that occurred from 1822 through 1930 and Black victim homicides between 1986 and 1995 in communities with lower percentages of votes for explicitly racist and segregationist presidential candidates Strom Thurmond in 1948 and George Wallace in 1968. "Such voting is symbolic of a change in racial politics and this study suggests that when White populations reject the agenda of racial dominance, legacies of historical racial violence can shift," Ward explained.[7]

The recognition that the effects of historical racial violence can be attenuated led Ward to focus on "memory work—the various ways we construct national memory and national identity." It includes both physical markers, such as monuments, statues, and plaques, and more interactive endeavors, such as museum exhibitions, storytelling, and theater.

> *These represent moments of refusing to look away, of lifting the "veil of oblivion" that has been so central to neglecting legacies of racial terror.*—Geoff K. Ward

Ward sees the potential for memory work to counter "willful ignorance" of history with an "intentionality about engaging who, in fact, we are, have been, and how we've gotten here, so that we might begin to change our national identity and shape a more inclusive vision of a collective future."

Exposing the Illusion That the Past Is Behind Us

Memory work fosters an acknowledgment of how much society continues to be influenced by the past. With that shared understanding, Ward said, it is possible to "think differently and to work differently together to change these dynamics."

Two research examples illustrate how relevant the past remains.

Lynching in the Past, Black Victim Homicide in the Present

The connection between a history of lynching and Black victim homicide, explained Ward, has much to do with the concept of legal estrangement, "the distrust of the state to provide protection and recourse." Police were invariably implicated in lynchings, either because they participated directly or because they aided and abetted others by withholding protection or failing to investigate the crime. This has often led people in communities with a history of lynching to settle disputes themselves, rather than to seek police intervention. Coupled with easy access to weapons, lethal violence has often been the result.

As evidence of an increased willingness to confront the past, Ward cited the memory work being done by a number of police departments across the country. By admitting to their role in this history of racial terror, they are acknowledging the legitimacy of the distrust built up over generations and seeking to build new relationships with Black communities.[8]

The hope of this memory work is that it gives police more perspective on the problem of structural racism and offers Black people and other populations reason to trust and cooperate with police. To be legitimate, the process must also include White people in the community. "We need White residents to understand the role White communities have played in corrupting the rule of law, and then to think critically about roles on juries or using 911 as a distress call when they feel uncomfortable," Ward emphasized. "We all need to process this historical trauma together and think about how we're all impacted by it and how our contemporary dynamics are connected to this long history of over-policing and under-protection."

Lynching in the Past, Corporal Punishment in the Present

In another example of the pull of history, an analysis of 11 southern states by Ward and colleagues found that the odds that a child, especially a Black child, will be subjected to corporal punishment in school increase significantly with every additional lynching that has occurred in the local county.[9] Ward suspects this reflects, in part, a continued desensitization toward violence against Black people in these areas.

He noted that leaders in post-apartheid South Africa are similarly coming to terms with the failure of their transitional justice process to address the dehumanization central to that racist structure, which is evident in enduring disregard for human rights. He and his coauthors also speculated that Black parents in areas with histories of lynching may allow schools to corporally punish their children, thinking it might later protect them outside school, where misbehavior "could prove fatal or extremely costly." The thinking, he said, is that if a child's relatively minor transgressions in school are corrected severely, he or she will be compliant as a young adult and more likely to follow the rules, and so be spared serious consequences at the hands of police, the courts, or others in the streets. The irony, said Ward, is that the evidence suggests the opposite: Corporal punishment is an adverse childhood experience that contributes to poor behavioral and other health outcomes in the future.

The Value of Memory Work

As a key example of memory work, memorial museums "use commemoration and education to seed understanding and deeper commitment to human rights and civil rights in post-conflict environments," said Ward. The Hiroshima Peace Memorial Museum in Japan, the Auschwitz-Birkenau Memorial and Museum in Poland, and the Apartheid Museum in South Africa are international examples. Domestic examples include the Legacy Museum and National Memorial for Peace and Justice in Montgomery, Ala., the U.S. Holocaust Memorial Museum in Washington, and the Mississippi Civil Rights Museum in Jackson, Miss.

Ward explored the notion of museum as intervention in an exhibition he curated for the Mildred Lane Kemper Art Museum at Washington University. The exhibition, *Truths and Reckonings: The Art of Transformative Racial Justice*, housed in the museum's teaching gallery, created a "pop-up" memorial museum, with the stated aim "to facilitate understanding and commemoration of this haunting presence of the past and encourage greater commitment to transformative racial justice."[10] The exhibition mixed works of art with historical objects, such as newspaper articles (e.g., *The Weekly Caucasian*, a White supremacist newspaper published between 1866 and 1875 in Missouri's "Little Dixie" region), photographs (including "lynching parties"), illustrations from pamphlets and magazines, and other artifacts. Ward has found that the items in the exhibit allow people to be less defensive and more open to conversations about the persistence of structural racism. The exhibition also served as a basis for discussions with local police that enabled participants to reflect together on a shared history. He noted that viewers repeatedly said that they knew nothing about this history and had never been exposed to it in their education—still another example of the "veil of oblivion."

Ward emphasized the many forms that memory work can take. Along with monuments and historical markers, heritage preservation can address the erasure of Black history and the histories of other people of color. "These interventions through commemorative work help us address the differential valuation of human beings or the scaling of bodies along racial lines," Ward remarked, "with some valued as more meaningful, more important, and more human than others" (see Chapter 1). He cited the preservation of an historical Black cemetery as an example. "The work of preserving that space and honoring the lives interred there has broader implications for how we relate to each other today and for our development of a greater ability to value and dignify each life equally."

> *People say we can't change the past. But we can and must change the representation and the meaning of the past in the present and future.*
> —Geoff K. Ward

Place Matters, History Matters

As evidence that the influence of history endures, one need look no further than the persistent racial discrimination that has characterized housing and real estate policy and practice over the last century. Two broad principles must be at the forefront when the subject is structural racism and how to address it, according to Ohio State University city and regional planning researcher Jason Reece.

The first is that *place matters*. "There is a tremendous geographical aspect to structural inequality and many structural barriers to opportunity manifest at a neighborhood scale," Reece noted. As a stark illustration, Reece compared the availability of resources in different Jackson, Miss., neighborhoods, based on data from the Child Opportunity Index. Developed by the Diversity Data Kids program at Brandeis University,[11] the index measures and maps quality education, safe housing, clean air, playgrounds, and other opportunity-based resources and indicators of child well-being. Its overarching finding is that disparities grow along with the proportion of Black residents. (For more on the Child Opportunity Index, see Chapter 9.) Neighborhoods characterized as having high or very high levels of opportunity on the index had the largest percentage of White children and the smallest percentage of Black children. The opposite was true of neighborhoods with low and very low opportunity scores. This recognition can inform and shift interventions, investment decisions, and policy levers "to open up access to different opportunities for folks in those communities," said Reece.

At the same time, *history matters*, as it is responsible for the variability of opportunity that is tied to place. The development of cities and regions was deeply racialized over the course of the 20th century, Reece stressed, and that racialization has significantly impacted how 21st-century communities look and operate and the level of trust community members have in the institutions and policies that affect their daily lives.

Racialized Policymaking

The exclusion of Black residents from neighborhoods of opportunity "has played a big role in shaping the 21st-century American city," said Reece. A form of historical trauma, the legacy has left an imprint that remains "front and center in the minds of folks who live in neighborhoods that have been on the receiving end of so many of these detrimental policies, eroding trust in the public sector and in the powers that guide urban development."

Two general types of policymaking influenced racialized community development: exclusion and segregation, and institutional disinvestment. This policymaking began in the early 20th century with racial zoning, a segregationist system that explicitly denied housing to certain racial groups. After the Supreme Court ruled in 1917 that such zoning violated the Fourteenth Amendment, alternative legislative routes were designed to accomplish much the same thing. Between 1920 and the 1950s, the use of restrictive covenants, which prohibited a property owner from selling or renting to people of a specified race, creed, or color, became a tool to segregate cities, according to Reece. Restrictive covenants were ultimately struck down by the courts as well, but the real estate sector worked with neighborhood associations to harass Black people out of specific neighborhoods or prevent them from ever moving in. (For more on how zoning influences access to housing, see Chapter 9.)

Redlining was another segregation strategy, and a particularly pernicious one. Beginning with the passage of the National Housing Act of 1934, redlining distinguished neighborhoods in which the Federal Housing Administration would insure mortgages from those in which it would not. The federal Home Owners Loan Corporation assessed properties in 239 cities and shared its maps with the Federal Housing Administration and with local lenders, banks, and planners. In practice, redlining restricted areas where Black people could purchase homes limited the opportunity for Black families to build wealth through property ownership and fostered underinvestment in neighborhoods in which they remained, typically as renters. Later, urban renewal and neighborhood demolition to "save" these neighborhoods further pushed Black people to under-resourced areas.

It was not just one policy or a single culprit, Reece stressed, but the interconnection of planning and built environment policies at the federal level with those at the local level where real estate, neighborhood association, and corporate interests align. And so, Reece concluded, "we have these very systemic discriminatory tools that get developed in cities, and the federal government—as part of the New Deal—embraces these tools and philosophies and adds a level of expansion and impact not seen before by bringing these practices to scale."

Policies are not neutral. They're shaped by values. Our housing development system and built environment, particularly in the 20th century, were shaped by vehemently racist values.

—Jason Reece

The conflict is ongoing. Wins toward equity are followed by a system realignment to achieve the same inequitable ends in other ways, said Reece, setting the stage for a fresh battle." Many policies appear race-neutral but in practice enable exclusionary land use practices that limit access to much of the housing market for people of color and lower-income people. As well, the suppression of property values in certain communities, reflecting decades of discriminatory practices, enables developers to flip homes far above their purchase prices as neighborhoods begin to gentrify, often forcing out long-time residents.

Nonetheless, there are signals of progress, noted Reece. He cited the Fair Housing Act of 1968, which prohibits discrimination in housing sales and rentals (including mortgages and housing assistance), as a fundamental shift in federal policy "unthinkable 20 years earlier." And present-day discussions about ending single-family zoning also herald new thinking about how to diversify communities.

Eliminating Structural Racism at the County Level

Cuyahoga County, Ohio, which includes Cleveland, adopted the elimination of structural racism as a primary policy goal for its public health agency. But Reece, who worked with the agency on its initiative, said "there was very little shared understanding of what that actually meant."

The PlaceMatters initiative for Cuyahoga County and the Cuyahoga County Board of Health was a multiyear planning process focused on the relationship between community conditions and community health. Recognizing that most people are unaware of the history of discrimination in the built environment, Reece and his team were asked to research and tell the story of Cuyahoga County through the lens of health equity. Working from historical artifacts, maps, and documents, including real estate assessor notes from the past, they prepared a report and conducted a series of public events to help stakeholders visualize the geography of discrimination.[12,13] Among the revelations:[14]

- An overlay of a 1940 redlining map with a 2010 map of infant mortality rates showed that infants in previously redlined neighborhoods were about 800% more likely to die than those in non-redlined neighborhoods.
- Life expectancy was an average of 12 years lower in neighborhoods that had been redlined.

• Foreclosures in Cuyahoga County during the 2008 housing crisis were among the highest in the nation, and the greatest number were in previously redlined areas. The legacy of discrimination had a direct influence on the subprime lending that took down the housing market.

Having an historical context helped county stakeholders recognize that small, short-term interventions would not remedy deep structural problems, and they began to consider changes that could help eradicate the racism at their core. Their report was "a critical piece of knowledge to help folks be able to talk about existing challenges," said Reece. "This ability to connect past to present in terms of policy has been really profound."

In a second Ohio-based project, Reece's team engaged with Franklin County Thrive, a community planning initiative, to address growing poverty in the region, which includes Columbus. Among participants were the United Way, a food bank, philanthropies, and representatives of the business, health, education, social service, and affordable housing sectors. Here, too, historical research demonstrated that the communities requiring the bulk of these services had historically faced discrimination through redlining and other practices. Results were presented to stakeholders through local media and on social media.

> *The data is jaw-dropping. There is always a bit of a gasp at the empirical connection, and at the strength of that connection, between historical discrimination and certain health outcomes.*
>
> —Jason Reece

In both PlaceMatters and Franklin County Thrives, stakeholders came to understand both the long-term nature of structural racism and the sustained effort that is needed for real change. As one person commented, "In order for us to solve the problems of today, it's essential that we understand how we got here."[15]

Reece recommends engaging with historical artifacts and documents as much as possible. While that can be traumatic for people who have experienced deep-seated discrimination, the language used in the original policy documents also reveals the true depths of bias. "There is value in airing the ugliness of these very racist statements that are in our policy documents and letting people see those," he argued.

The influence of past practices remains evident in the events that transformed American life in 2020. The pattern of COVID-19 outbreaks in Columbus, for example, closely tracked the pattern of redlining. "They're the miner's canary," said Reece, "the ones that are hit first and hit hardest." Likewise, the pattern of police shootings aligns with the location of redlined neighborhoods. "When we see incidents of police violence, it's often in many of these same spaces," he noted.

Expanding Young People's Understanding of History

The lack of knowledge among young people about the racial underpinnings of much of U.S. history troubles Reece: "Until we accept the fact that we've whitewashed much of our history and we fundamentally transform the way we're teaching history, this will continue to be a problem because we don't have that shared dialogue." Reece is committed to integrating this knowledge into school curricula.

To foster understanding about where they live, Reece and reporters from Columbus's local newspaper, *The Dispatch*, worked with high school students to research neighborhood history and its impact on current conditions. Like most people, the students had taken differences in neighborhood characteristics for granted without thinking more deeply about why a highway was located in a particular spot or why houses on one side were more distressed than on the other. "It has been an eye-opening process that has helped them think about the built environment and the social environment and make those connections," he said. (For more on expanding young people's understanding of the impact of history on health, see the Spotlight at the end of this chapter.)

Symbols, Stressors, and Black Emotional Health

It is not only the history of violence and discrimination but also the symbols and images of that history that damage the health of Black people today. In Mississippi, "if someone's great-great-great-grandfather fought in the Civil War, then that's blood, and blood has always been seen to be thicker than water," said Byron D'Andra Orey, a political scientist at Jackson State University. "And that's considered to be heritage." This principle is at the heart of the concept of "cultural conservatism" and concern that threats to Confederate symbols are threats to heritage.

"The epitome of cultural conservatism is the case of the Mississippi state flag," said Orey, which included the Confederate battle insignia in the upper left corner from 1894 until it was replaced in January 2021. For many years, it was the only state flag that retained a Confederate emblem. Those who supported it claimed to see it as a symbol of their heritage, while many others considered it a stark and divisive reminder of slavery. Orey cited a 2001 statewide survey by the Jackson, Miss., newspaper, *The Clarion Ledger*, which found that 76% of those for whom the flag represented slavery were Black, while 72% of those who saw it as a symbol of their heritage were White.[16] In an April 2001 referendum, 65% of Mississippians voted to keep the flag, a repudiation that motivated Orey to leave his faculty position at Jackson State and move to Nebraska.

When I see the flag, I see Dylan Roof who went into the church in Charleston, S.C., and killed those parishioners who were in prayer service. He'd been seen with this battle flag. I see the Ku Klux Klan. I see segregation. And I had to leave Mississippi because it was taking a mental toll on me.

—Byron D'Andra Orey

At the University of Nebraska, Orey connected with researchers in the field of biopolitics, the intersection of biology and political science. Orey developed knowledge and skills in biopolitics and began to think about the physiological impact of exposure to racist symbols. He returned to Jackson State just when a Black attorney, Carlos Moore, filed a lawsuit claiming that seeing the Mississippi flag had negatively affected him both physically and mentally. A judge ruled that Moore had not shown injury or harm,[17] and Orey decided it was time to put his biopolitics skills to work.

Detecting Emotional Response

To determine whether viewing the flag and other Confederate symbols has physiological effects, Orey and his team measured the galvanic skin response of Black people as they looked at these symbols. The electrical conductivity of skin changes when a person is exposed to emotionally charged images, events, or other stimuli. Galvanic skin response, resulting from sweating on the hands and feet, is an especially sensitive measure of emotional arousal. This response is controlled by the autonomic sympathetic nervous system that regulates unconscious physical actions (e.g., heart rate, digestion, respiration) and activates the fight-or-flight response. Orey's conclusion: Black people who viewed Confederate symbols did, indeed, display a greater galvanic skin response than when they viewed neutral images, such as a basket.[18]

The researchers also used electrocardiograms to measure changes in heart rate and ocular response to track the extent to which the viewer was actually looking at a Confederate symbol rather than something else in the photo. That kind of methodology makes it possible to collect evidence of emotional arousal and document the source of high blood pressure, heart disease, immune system suppression, sleep disorders, and other health problems associated with extended stimulation of the sympathetic nervous system.

Orey has conducted similar research on Black people's responses to images of traffic stops by police, while a colleague at the University of Michigan is collecting the same data from White people for comparison. Such research can be used "to educate the public that institutional racism and structural racism have an impact on health," he said. Along with incorporating that kind of information into school curricula to reach young people, mental health professionals are an important audience; they are often unaware of the cumulative trauma that Black people face and uncertain how to treat it.

Back to the Flag

Bills to change the Mississippi flag were repeatedly introduced in the legislature in the years since the 2001 referendum and never made it out of committee. But the increased attention to racial injustice in 2020 finally altered the climate. Young protesters, Black and White, lobbied for the change. Entertainers weighed in, as did a number of Mississippi-based companies. And Kylin Hill, a star football player at Mississippi State, threatened to leave the team if the flag was not changed.[19] These factors "made way for removal," said Orey. "It was not that we had these goodhearted legislators. They were really pressured."

On June 28, 2020, the Mississippi legislature passed a bill to remove the Confederate symbol, and it was subsequently signed by Governor Tate Reeves. The bill established a commission to create a new flag, and Mississippi voters chose the new design in the November election, with 73% approval. On January 11, 2021, the new flag was flown over the state Capitol for the first time, finally removing this symbol of historical violence and trauma from common view.

Building a Knowledge Base for Growth

The story of the Mississippi flag suggests that a community can reckon with long histories of racial violence and discrimination and in doing so can address the health outcomes and inequities that are the contemporary consequences (see the Prologue to this book). But as the contributors to this chapter have suggested, meaningful change requires a shared understanding of that history.

Adams County, Miss., borders the Mississippi River about two hours southwest of Jackson. The county seat, Natchez, is the oldest settlement on the river. Madeline England of the Mississippi State Department of Health describes it as "a very small, rural southern Mississippi town with an industry mostly based on heritage tourism, especially antebellum mansions." (Adams County is one of 30 RWJF Sentinel Communities that inform the Culture of Health Action Framework.)

Mirroring a national trend over the past few decades, a recognition has emerged that Black history in Adams County is underrepresented in historical buildings preservation and physical infrastructure as well as in less tangible forms of preservation and cultural heritage. In 2016, Natchez celebrated its tricentennial with a yearlong series of arts and cultural events that included discussions about what residents wanted their city to look like in the future. A downtown master plan was developed and over the next few years, a number of efforts were made to acknowledge the past. A local community organization, the Friends of the Forks of the Road Society, installed a plaque at Forks of the Road, the site of the second largest slave market in the South from 1833 until 1863; the National Park Service has taken ownership of the site and plans to do more there in the future.

In another effort, the Historic Natchez Foundation used a grant from the National Park Service African American Civil Rights Grant Program to launch the Adams County Civil Rights Project to study and commemorate Black history. To understand the connections between this project and the health of area residents, community-led committees conducted an 18-month health impact assessment. The assessment was administered by the Mississippi State Department of Health, with funding from the Health Impact Project, a collaboration of RWJF and the Pew Charitable Trusts.

The mixed-methods research design used community engagement, local and state case studies, and literature review to explore three questions:[20]

- How does the process of publicly identifying and interpreting civil rights sites impact the health and well-being of Adams County residents?
- How does transforming the built environment through historical preservation impact the health and well-being of Adams County residents?
- How might place-based educational tools for local civil rights history impact the health and well-being of Adams County residents, particularly youth?

Project partners presented to local government and organized focus groups, public and private meetings, and multiple community events to gather a wide range of input. From the beginning, the Black community was clear that White residents should be a part of the process, not only to bring people together but also, importantly, to drive accountability. Believing that the White community lacked historical knowledge, "they wanted people to confront that history," England said. Though a true reconciliation effort was beyond the project scope, members of the White community were active participants.

The project team found that if community members were asked a very straightforward question—for example, "what sites represent civil rights to you in our community?"—people would highlight high-profile, often traumatic, one-time events, such as a murder or an incident of cross burning. The team labeled these events, which tended to focus on White control and violence and Black victimization, "acute historical trauma." That focus often results in a memorial or monument, which becomes little more than a destination for White tourists, England explained: "This can reinforce the existing status quo rather than answer questions about who should be telling the story, how this story is told, and who benefits from the story."

People wanted "to bring in the much deeper, daily lived experience," said England, "and tell more stories about the families and lives of these people and not just about their murders. They wanted to celebrate Black people and Black heroes." The team decided to change its approach and to seek multi-layered insights about "chronic historical trauma," which is often overlooked. They began by asking different questions aimed at compiling a more comprehensive story of civil rights history. For example, community members were asked how civil rights played into the evolution of a specific neighborhood. "The conversation became substantively different and community engagement became a lot more meaningful," said England. "We were able to gather stories about chronic historical trauma and structural racism and actually get into a series of inequities that are still very much a part of the community today." As a result, community members began to develop a collective understanding of how structural racism had become embedded in the community over centuries.

The health impact assessment report issued in 2019 included recommendations to:[21]

- Support education on local civil rights for youth in schools and youth groups.
- Develop a cross-sector strategy and infrastructure for cultural equity for community development, economic diversity, entrepreneurship, and outcome measurement.
- Build collective efficacy and counter-narratives around civil rights history.
- Develop an interactive People's Civil Rights Trail.
- Coordinate research on historical inequities at the neighborhood level to increase understanding of contemporary health inequities.

Action on these recommendations has been constrained by the pandemic, which has shifted local and health department priorities, and by a lack of clarity over ongoing ownership of the project. But progress is evident: The Task Force for Tourism, Ingenuity and Diversity, established by the new mayor of Natchez, is overseeing development of a monument to the United States Colored Troops[22] (many of whom came from Natchez) and working to preserve and recognize Black historical sites. England believes the work has made a substantive difference in community knowledge about health inequities, the role of history, and the long-term damage both can do unless they receive adequate attention. She acknowledged, however, that it is too soon to measure its health impact.

Because of structural racism, we've created these divisions that we don't even see—especially the White community does not see the depth of inequity.

With the health impact assessment we have begun to develop a knowledge base that we can grow together.

—Madeline England

A Final Word

A history of racist violence tied to slavery, lynching, and other brutalities continues to shape experiences of violence and the health status of Black people. Likewise, long-standing discriminatory practices in housing and real estate remain influences on contemporary segregation and the resources and opportunities available in primarily Black neighborhoods.

Understanding these connections is critical to alleviating contemporary harms, yet many of them have been obscured or ignored altogether. The controversy raised in some school districts by the use of the curriculum from the *New York Times Magazine*'s 1619 Project highlights the challenges of incorporating this history into K–12 education.[23,24,25] While some school systems have adopted the curriculum, which puts the consequences of slavery and the struggle of Black Americans to realize the ideals of democracy at the center of the American story, others have resisted its depiction of racism as a founding principle. (For more on the 1619 Project, see Chapter 1.)

To move in a new direction we all must learn the lessons of the past and apply this collective understanding to heal our neighborhoods and communities. Young people—with their curiosity, enthusiasm, and energy—must be given the knowledge, tools, and opportunities to take these lessons into the future. This is how we can, as Geoff K. Ward advocates, "change the representation and the meaning of the past" and bend the historical arc away from violence and toward justice and equity.

Spotlight

Youth Changing the Narrative on Health

Cristy Johnston Limón, MBA, Former Executive Director, Youth Speaks

How can young people contribute to changing the narrative in order to link the health challenges in communities of color to a history of violence and discrimination? Youth Speaks is helping them find the answers.

Founded in San Francisco's Mission District in 1996 to empower young people from underresourced and underrepresented communities, Youth Speaks is the largest youth poetry nonprofit organization in the United States. The organization works with young people who are disconnected from civic life and lack opportunities for arts education and other youth development activities, said former executive director Cristy Johnston Limón. Limón described participants as urban youth of color, ages 13 to 19, from low-income communities that historically have been "silenced, marginalized, or otherwise excluded from fully participating in defining their own narratives." Through storytelling and poetry drawn from their lived experience, these young people "learn that they can and do shape the world around them," observed Limón.

> *Youth discover that they have agency and can use their voices, their words, and their actions to effect positive change.*
>
> —Cristy Johnston Limón

One of Youth Speaks signature programs is The Bigger Picture, developed in collaboration with the Center for Vulnerable Populations at the University of California, San Francisco. An arts-based public health literacy program, The Bigger Picture was initially designed to increase youth awareness of the complex factors behind the high rates of type 2 diabetes in Black and Latino communities

Cristy Johnston Limón, *Spotlight* In: *Necessary Conversations*. Edited by: Alonzo L. Plough, Oxford University Press. © Robert Wood Johnson Foundation 2022. DOI: 10.1093/oso/9780197641477.003.0013

so they can "move from being targets of metabolic risk to agents of change," as Limón described it. More recently, The Bigger Picture has expanded its focus to confront the disproportionate impact of police violence, climate change, and COVID-19 on the health of communities of color.

Over a lifetime, 40% of all Americans are at risk of developing type 2 diabetes, but that figure rises to 50% among non-Hispanic Black women and Hispanic men and women.[1] Young people are unaware of how historically discriminatory practices in housing, education, healthcare, and the physical environment can influence these statistics. "They have been blamed for making bad choices," said Limón, "rather than considering the larger environmental and social determinants of health." As an example, television advertising for unhealthy snacks and sugary beverages targeted to Black viewers increased 50% between 2013 and 2017.[2]

The Bigger Picture, which has won health and media/film awards, uses a combination of classroom work, mini-documentaries, and social media to educate and engage young people. Curricula provide both historical and current data and opportunities for stories and lived experience to consider how food deserts, food insecurity, sugary beverages, and marketing contribute to the epidemic of diabetes in these communities.

"We use the arts to facilitate youth to think about, imagine, feel, and taste what their neighborhoods are like and what their lived experience is in order to frame a different analysis of the causes of type 2 diabetes," said Limón. By asking questions about the presence or absence of fast-food restaurants, playgrounds, liquor stores, farmers markets, and other features of their neighborhoods, systemic environmental disparities in access to healthy food and physical activity become apparent. These young participants write about their own experience, which then becomes the content for poems and videos that are shared throughout the community, spreading awareness and clarity.

The University of California, Berkeley, evaluated the model during the 2019–20 school year at six public high schools in San Francisco: three receiving the intervention, three serving as comparison schools. (During the pandemic the program has been presented online.) Initial results indicate that the intervention "advances a Culture of Health by influencing the mindsets and expectations of the youth and creates a sense of community and civic engagement among them," reported Limón.

Fair Housing, Equitable Communities

Dolores Acevedo-Garcia, PhD, Professor of Human Development and Social Policy Director, Institute for Child, Youth and Family Policy, Heller School for Social Policy and Management, Brandeis University

Solomon Greene, JD, MCP, Senior Fellow, Research to Action Lab and Metropolitan Housing and Communities Policy Center, Urban Institute

Demetria McCain, Esq., Former President, Inclusive Communities Project

Nick Mitchell-Bennett, MA, Executive Director, come dream. come build.

Primus Wheeler, MS, Executive Director, Jackson Medical Mall Foundation*

Where people live—their homes, neighborhoods, and regions—is a prime contributor to health and, as the previous chapter makes clear, is often heavily influenced by historical discrimination. This chapter examines local and regional strategies to strengthen communities and improve the affordability, availability, and quality of housing and neighborhoods for low-income Black and Latino families. These are the populations most likely to have been excluded from

---

* Demetria McCain participated in the Robert Wood Johnson Foundation's Sharing Knowledge conference in 2020 in her role as president of the Inclusive Communities Project. Any comments attributed to Ms. McCain in this chapter were made prior to her service at the U.S. Department of Housing and Urban Development (HUD) beginning in September 2021. Any quotes or insights attributed to Ms. McCain in this chapter reflect her views as an expert on fair housing, and do not reflect the views or positions of HUD or the U.S. government.

Dolores Acevedo-Garcia, Solomon Greene, Demetria McCain, Nick Mitchell-Bennett, and Primus Wheeler, *Fair Housing, Equitable Communities* In: *Necessary Conversations*. Edited by: Alonzo L. Plough, Oxford University Press. © Robert Wood Johnson Foundation 2022. DOI: 10.1093/oso/9780197641477.003.0014

neighborhoods of opportunity and to lack meaningful choice in their housing decisions.

Chapter contributors offer historical and contemporary perspectives on equitable communities, the affordable housing crisis, and the public policies that can generate needed change. Brandeis University professor Dolores Acevedo-Garcia describes deep disparities across the nation's neighborhoods as she presents findings from the Child Opportunity Index. The Urban Institute's Solomon Greene addresses the potential risks and benefits of zoning and land use reforms while fair housing advocate Demetria McCain of the Inclusive Communities Project describes ways to ensure that people have genuine housing choice. Nick Mitchell-Bennett, at come dream. come build. (cdcb, the organization's standard capitalization) draws on his experience as a nonprofit housing developer to explain how very low-income people on the southern U.S. border can build home equity.

Finally, in a Spotlight, Primus Wheeler, executive director of the Jackson Medical Mall Foundation, describes this innovative enterprise, which combines healthcare, community development (including affordable home ownership), arts and culture, and innovation and technology to renew and strengthen a Jackson, Miss., community.

Key Elements of an Equitable Community

One lesson from the previous chapter is that "place matters." Where a child grows up, where teens begin to assert their independence, and where adults live and work has a big impact on their physical, mental, emotional, and social health. But the resources and opportunities available across neighborhoods throughout the United States vary widely, depriving far too many of the prospects for a fulfilling and satisfying life.

Here, a researcher and an advocate consider what it will take to change that so everyone can live in an equitable community. Solomon Greene from the Urban Institute described an equitable community as one that includes all elements necessary for social, economic, physical, and mental well-being and that serves as a "launching pad" to propel all who live there toward opportunity. It is also democratically governed and takes affirmative steps to reduce inequalities. But even meeting all of those benchmarks does not ensure equity, emphasized Greene, explaining that communities are "fluid, and how we define a community can actually turn an equitable one into an exclusive one."

An equitable community recognizes its place within the broader community or region—for example by shouldering its fair share of affordable housing

*and not hoarding opportunities[1] and making it impossible for others to ac-
cess them or to remain in the community as it thrives.*

—Solomon Greene

To be truly equitable, a community must be diverse, providing a home to residents
across income levels and representing a mix of ages, races, and ethnicities, in the
view of Demetria McCain of the Inclusive Communities Project. Universally accessible amenities are also essential (for example, parks open at times available
to people with different work hours), as well as affordable retail, equity in the
schools, and community safety for everyone. "I do not call a community equitable if it is diverse but doesn't have services that are accessible and positive for
everybody," McCain stressed. "It's got to have both."

The Impact of Place on Opportunity

Achieving the ideal of true equity across communities requires, first, an understanding of how, where, and to what extent communities differ in the prospects
afforded to its residents. The Child Opportunity Index offers that understanding. The index measures and maps the quality of neighborhood resources
and conditions conducive to healthy child development across the United Sates.
Developed in 2014 with funding from RWJF[2,3] and the W.K. Kellogg Foundation,
the index is produced by diversitydatakids.org at Brandeis University's Institute
for Child, Youth, and Family Policy, led by Acevedo-Garcia. Version 2.0 of the
index launched in 2020.

Children's neighborhoods influence their health and educational outcomes,
play an important role in shaping their expectations for their own futures, and
impact long-term outcomes, such as socioeconomic mobility and health and life
expectancy. The ability to choose the neighborhood that offers the best opportunities for children is a civil rights issue, argued Acevedo-Garcia.

*Children should have access to a good quality of life in their neighborhoods
and have the right to an enjoyable childhood experience.*

—Dolores Acevedo-Garcia

The index captures the complexity of neighborhood-based resources for
healthy child development in all 72,000 U.S. census tracts.[4] It is based on 29
indicators of child well-being in three domains—education, health and environment, and social and economic. Among the indicators are access to quality
early childhood education, high-quality schools, green space, healthy food, and
toxin-free environments, and rates of employment, poverty, and homeownership. Data are from 2010 and 2015, the most recent available.

The index allows the quality of children's neighborhoods to be compared within and between cities, regions, and states, or nationwide. A summary Child Opportunity Score is calculated for each neighborhood from 1 (lowest level of neighborhood opportunity) to 100 (highest level of neighborhood opportunity). In addition, neighborhoods are sorted into five Childhood Opportunity Levels: very low, low, moderate, high, or very high, with each containing 20% of the U.S. population under the age of 18.

Some findings from these rankings:[5]

- Levels of child opportunity tend to be lower in the South.
- Among the 100 largest metropolitan areas, Fresno, Calif., has the lowest Child Opportunity Score (20), while Madison, Wis., and San Jose, Calif., have the highest (83).
- Opportunity varies greatly between metropolitan areas. For example, Memphis, Tenn., has a Child Opportunity Score of 34 while Minneapolis, Minn., is at 80.

Across the 100 largest metropolitan areas:

- Life expectancy in very low opportunity neighborhoods is 75 years compared with 82 years in very high opportunity neighborhoods.
- At age 35, a child from a low-income family (25th percentile of income distribution) in a very low opportunity neighborhood will have an average income of $29,268. At the same age, a child from a similar low-income family in a very high opportunity neighborhood will have an average income of $45,500.

Within metropolitan areas, the differences between neighborhoods can be huge—larger, in fact, than between metropolitan areas. Often, within a single metropolitan area, very low opportunity neighborhoods have scores of 2 or 3, while very high opportunity neighborhoods have scores greater than 90. To illustrate the vast chasm, Acevedo-Garcia presented data from two neighborhoods in Jackson, Miss, which has an overall score of 41. In one, only 2% of families live in poverty, 11% of teachers have less than three years teaching experience, and less than 2% of the housing units are vacant. In a neighborhood about three miles away, almost half of families live in poverty, one-third of teachers have less than three years of teaching experience, and 13% of the housing units are vacant.

The strongest predictors of a neighborhood's level of child opportunity are the race and ethnicity of its residents. In Jackson less than 2% of White children live in very low opportunity neighborhoods, compared to 35% of Black children, while 40% of White children and 6% of Black children live in very high opportunity neighborhoods. Jackson is not unique in this regard, added Acevedo-Garcia. "That is a sad pattern that we see across the U.S. In almost every metro area the neighborhoods of White children have a higher score than the overall score and those of Black and Hispanic children have a lower score than the overall."

The opportunities available to children as they develop have profound implications both for their own future and for society in general. The long-term effects of growing up in poorly resourced neighborhoods not only limit individual health and economic opportunities but are also injurious to families and communities. Ensuring that communities become more equitable requires concerted attention to the laws, norms, and practices that influence neighborhood characteristics and housing choices.

Harnessing the Power of Zoning

"Buy land, they're not making it anymore," said Mark Twain. Agreeing with Twain's tongue-in-cheek observation, researcher Solomon Greene has turned his attention to zoning and other land use regulations that shape what can be built, and where. All 50 states have legislation that empowers municipalities or counties to enact their own zoning laws to regulate residential and commercial development.[6] While Greene acknowledged that zoning often gets "a bad rap" because it can be used to exclude people by race, ethnicity, religion, or income, it can also shape a community in positive ways. For example, zoning can contribute to environmental sustainability by keeping growth within boundaries and protecting wetlands. It can also help cities "right-size" based on their resources and resident preferences—for example, by ensuring that housing development does not overwhelm school size or road traffic capacity.

But in practice, zoning and other policies have often curbed the ability to meet local needs, especially for affordable housing or indeed any new housing at all. Zoning laws and other regulations that were explicitly or implicitly racist have been struck down over time by Supreme Court decisions and civil rights laws (for more on this history, see Chapter 8). While local governments no longer explicitly refer to race in their zoning laws and decisions, the status quo has been preserved by requirements for large lots or single-family homes and discretionary review processes that emphasize "community aesthetics and character," said Greene. Calls for local autonomy can result in strong opposition to new building projects from incumbent homeowners, effectively holding back affordable housing.

Mitigating Negative Zoning Impact

Greene described several state and local reform efforts that could mitigate the negative impact of zoning restrictions and increase the amount and spread of affordable housing.

Increase Density

Local governments can allow developers to build larger buildings, build over the full lot rather than requiring setbacks, or build more units on a given plot of land. Density can also be increased by building smaller units on smaller parcels. "Tiny homes" and "accessory dwelling units," which became popular during the pandemic as offices and home-schooling spaces, are examples of building smaller to increase density.

Cut the Red Tape

"Time is money" is a development industry truism. Lengthy, duplicative review processes and complicated legal and financing requirements take time and drive up building project costs. A "powerful reform," Greene said, "is allowing multifamily housing as a right." Zoning codes that explicitly permit multifamily housing allow developers to proceed with a code-compliant project without extensive discretionary review. Other reforms include one-stop permit shopping, rather than having to apply for multiple permits from different government entities, and expedited approvals for affordable housing.

Reduce Requirements

Reducing unnecessary and redundant requirements will also decrease building costs and design constraints, making affordable housing projects more feasible. For example, parking space requirements can be superfluous in cities with good public transportation, senior housing projects, and places seeking to promote walkability.[7] Such requirements take space, must be worked into the building design, and can add substantially to construction costs yet may be entirely unnecessary. Easing restrictions on the use of modular or manufactured housing is another strategy to increase the feasibility of affordable developments.

Boost Affordability

Boosting affordability is essential yet too often overlooked, Greene emphasized, because building more units and lifting regulatory restrictions will not by themselves meet the needs of low-income families who have been shut out of the housing market. Two other strategies can help increase affordability, according to his research: public subsidies and various types of inclusionary zoning policies. Subsidizing rents, financing housing trust funds, and providing tax credits to developers who build low-income housing are all mechanisms for putting public money into housing with the stipulation that it be kept affordable, as defined locally. Inclusionary zoning—ordinances that require or encourage some percentage of new housing units to be made available to people with limited incomes—"is a step in the right direction that has led to an increase in the number of affordable units at low to no cost to taxpayers," said Greene.

Approaches vary, as do the outcomes they produce. One strategy is requiring "in-lieu fees" in which developers pay into an affordable housing trust fund, which a specialized developer can then draw on to build affordable units in a low-cost community. Although this increases the number of affordable units, it also tends to perpetuate segregation. Alternatively, developers can be required to include affordable units on-site, which brings lower-income families into neighborhoods that have greater opportunity. But this strategy raises building costs, resulting in fewer affordable units. With voluntary inclusionary zoning, developers are not required to build affordable units but they will receive concessions, such as an allowance to add floors, if they do.

Research suggests the importance of designing policies carefully. "Inclusionary zoning, when done right, seems to be a net positive from an affordable housing standpoint," Greene noted, adding some caveats. It works best in high-growth communities, not in slow markets where home and land prices are declining or the population is decreasing. Also, while inclusionary projects can meet the needs of low- to moderate-income families, they are rarely oriented to the poorest people, those with physical disabilities, or other households that face the highest barriers to finding affordable housing.

Risk Along with Reform

Greene cited three main risks with current reform efforts. First, since many reforms are directed specifically at affordability, they may not address racial disparities: "This can mean that communities of color disproportionately bear the brunt of up-zoning [increasing density]. It can lead to counterproductive divides between those advocating for fair housing, civil rights, and equity and those who just want to see housing built." A move away from subsidies and tenant protections in favor of more market-based solutions, such as zoning and land use reforms, is a second concern to Greene. These reforms are, he said, "deregulatory in nature, and a blanket endorsement of deregulation as a housing strategy could have a chilling effect on healthy housing, environmental, and other protective regulations that we do want in place."

Finally, "local politics can be poorly suited to meeting broader housing needs," Greene believes, "and we may need to take decision-making to a higher level."

Decision-Making at the Regional or State Level

A few states, including California, Oregon, Utah, and Virginia, have adopted statewide zoning reform. More commonly, incorporated municipalities zone within their own borders and counties zone for the rest of county land. Allowing each locality to set its own rules leads to the current system in which localities focus on their own interests to the exclusion of neighboring communities and certain groups of people who want to move in. Often the goal is to attract residents and businesses who will bring in more tax revenue and consume fewer municipal services. This protection of individual community interests leads to an undersupply of housing in general and a significant undersupply of affordable housing.

New Jersey has been a notable exception to this trend as a result of the Mount Laurel Doctrine, which originates from two cases (1975 and 1983) in which the state Supreme Court ruled that land use regulations against affordable housing were unconstitutional.[8] Many consider the Mount Laurel Doctrine to be one of the most important civil rights cases since *Brown v. Board of Education* desegregated schools in 1954. In response, the New Jersey legislature enacted the Fair Housing Act, which mandates the distribution of affordable housing equitably across municipalities. In 2013, Princeton sociologist Douglas S. Massey, PhD, and colleagues determined that the result was "the creation of 60,000 homes for low- and moderate-income working families, with another 40,000 units in the pipeline," according to a *New York Times* report.[9,10]

> *From a racial equity standpoint, it is going to be important, if not essential, for states and the federal government to play a more active role addressing the tendency of some local governments to exclude.*
>
> —Solomon Greene

Greene also addressed planning in regions connected by jobs, commuting patterns, and housing. Unlike transportation authorities, which are required to operate as regional entities to secure federal funding, housing has received little attention at a regional level. Greene believes that should be the future of sound planning and wants the federal government to support a more regional approach. The Obama administration's Sustainable Communities Initiative, which offered grants for regional sustainability planning that integrated environmental, land use, and housing goals, was a step in that direction. One element, the Fair Housing and Equity Assessment, was essentially a regional fair housing plan, according to Greene, but Congress cut funding for its implementation, undermining action.

Beyond Zoning Reform

Sometimes more regulation, such as just-cause eviction statutes and rent stabili-zation codes, is needed to create an equitable community. During the pandemic, eviction moratoria proved critical to reducing the harms of involuntary house-hold moves. "We need to be real about which regulations are advancing health equity and which are hurting it," Greene observed.

Strategies to address persistent discrimination—from limiting the use of biased algorithms for lending decisions to creating more affordable mortgage products for buyers of color without strong credit scores—are vital to curb seg-regation and advance racial equity. Enforcing existing fair housing laws would also give teeth to that commitment. "There's a lot we can do beyond zoning reforms to improve racial equity in housing," said Greene. (For a look at one strategy to expand affordable housing and strengthen communities, see the Spotlight at the end of this chapter.)

Advancing Housing Choice in Dallas

Along with regulatory changes, and planning at multiple government levels, the federal Housing Choice Voucher Program (often referred to as "Section 8") can improve opportunities for low-income people and people of color seeking affordable housing. Section 8 vouchers, available to very low-income families, the elderly, and people with disabilities, can be applied toward rent in any loca-tion that meets program health and safety requirements, if the landlord agrees to accept them. Participants pay 30% of their income toward rent, with the re-mainder paid directly to the landlord by the federal government. A family may also apply its voucher to a home purchase if it is approved by the local public housing authority (the agency that administers federal aid provided by the U.S. Department of Housing and Urban Development [HUD] at the local level).

The Dallas Housing Authority administers 14,000 Section 8 housing vouchers. Voucher holders, who are about 85% Black, are most likely to live in areas with long-standing patterns of housing discrimination and limited oppor-tunity. This is clearly documented in maps that overlay the location of voucher holders with maps depicting historically redlined areas, low scores on the Child Opportunity Index, and high scores on the U.S. Treasury Department's CDFI Distress Index (a measure of community disadvantage related to the federal Community Development Financial Institutions Fund program). (See Chapter 8 for more on racialized policymaking.)

Many families would like to use their vouchers to move to higher-opportunity neighborhoods, but there are often obstacles to doing so. As president of the

Inclusive Communities Project in Dallas, which works directly with Section 8 voucher holders, Demetria McCain is committed to helping families overcome those obstacles. "We are an affordable fair housing group and our advocacy work is to push back any barriers our families experience in moving," said McCain. Obstacles often include landlords who require tenant income of three times the full rent, rather than three times the tenant's portion of the rent, or unreasonable housing authority time limits for tenants to find suitable housing. Inclusive Communities engages in advocacy, policy work, and direct services to fulfill its three-part mission:

- Create and maintain racially, ethnically, and economically inclusive communities.
- Expand affordable fair housing opportunities for low-income families in the region.
- Seek redress for policies and practices that perpetuate the effects of racial and ethnic segregation and discrimination.

As evidence for the significance of neighborhood, McCain drew on the research of Harvard University economist Raj Chetty, PhD, and colleagues on the federal Moving to Opportunity experiment. Their studies showed that adult outcomes are shaped by the neighborhoods in which they grew up and that moving to neighborhoods with greater opportunity can be a long-term benefit to children.[11]

But moving to better opportunity doesn't just happen. Inclusive Communities provides "housing mobility" services to people who want to use vouchers "to move outside racially isolated high poverty areas. It's called the 'housing choice voucher program,' but what is choice if they're not informed?" McCain asked.[†]

Recognizing that the housing authority sometimes steers families to places they don't want to live, counselors join them at housing authority briefings to explain their rights and make sure they understand that they can use their vouchers in Dallas County and all six adjacent counties. They also offer one-on-one counseling to assess family housing needs and preferences, suggest cities and communities that might interest them, and identify landlords who accept vouchers. A specialized website provides more information about the resources and amenities available in each neighborhood.

[†] Ms. McCain participated in the *Sharing Knowledge* conference in 2020 in her role as president of the Inclusive Communities Project. Any comments attributed to Ms. McCain in this chapter were made prior to her service at HUD beginning in September 2021. Any quotes or insights attributed to Ms. McCain in this chapter do not reflect the views or positions of HUD or the U.S. government.

The organization also addresses issues related to the federal Low-Income Housing Tax Credit program, which is now the source of most public funding to build new housing.[12] Developers receive tax credits for building or renovating housing targeted to low-income households and sell those credits to investors, generating equity to fund a project. By federal law, landlords of low-income tax credit complexes may not turn away voucher holders.

But that's only if the project gets built. Too often, neighborhood groups will lobby at meetings where a developer is seeking approval to build affordable housing and create fear. "You have these voices saying 'no' to City Council and you don't have any voices saying 'yes,'" McCain observed. Through its Voices for Opportunity program Inclusive Communities encourages families to at-tend and speak up at meetings, sending the message, "I'm a real person and stop talking about me like I'm the boogie man." Said McCain, "It's very empowering for those families and it makes a difference to them." Whether it makes a differ-ence with the decision-makers or influences their ultimate vote is not clear, she acknowledged. "But it can turn down the heat in the room a bit."

> *There is lots of discrimination. Nobody wants to take voucher holders, and while there is lots of new development everybody is kicking out people with low incomes.*
>
> —Demetria McCain

Texas is one of two states (along with Indiana) that pre-empt cities and counties from passing ordinances to stop landlords from discriminating against people based on their source of income.[13] That allows landlords to turn away qualified rental applicants who would be using a Section 8 voucher. Landlords are increasingly likely to do just that. A 2020 survey conducted by the organiza-tion found that only 7% of Dallas-area landlords accepted vouchers in the areas studied, a drop from an earlier survey in 2017, when they were accepted by 12% of landlords.

Inclusive Communities is tracking two bills in the Texas legislature: One would eliminate pre-emption of local voucher discrimination ordinances while the other would affirmatively prohibit voucher discrimination through the state's Fair Housing Act, overriding local ordinances. Although she acknowledged that passage of the legislation is an uphill battle, McCain called for a deeper com-mitment to racial equity in housing. Like Greene, she highlighted the impor-tance of inclusionary zoning, with the building of units sized to meet the needs of families.

Housing voucher subsidies that reflect realistic market rents in a local, ZIP-code–based area can remove another barrier for people seeking housing options. In Dallas, such subsidies have been in place since Inclusive Communities settled a case with HUD in 2011. McCain also sees a growing interest from White middle-income allies in the possibility of changing local policies to support fair housing.

Honoring Choice, Building Wealth in the Rio Grande Valley

Just as Inclusive Communities focuses on improving lives in the Black communities the agency serves, another Texas organization far from Dallas supports housing choice and change for low- and very low-income Latino families. The city of Brownsville lies at the southernmost tip of Texas near the Gulf Coast and just across the Rio Grande from Mexico, about 550 miles south of Dallas. It is a stark landscape. "We are 4,000 square miles of low-lying," said Nick Mitchell-Bennett, executive director of come dream. come build. (cdcb), a Brownsville-based community housing development organization that has served the Rio Grande Valley since 1974. "We are *not* a valley. There isn't a hill in sight. We are a river delta just like the Mississippi Delta. It's low lying and it floods when it rains. And we have lots and lots of hurricanes."

The main mission of cdcb is to help families in this border region, where the population is about 94% Latino and poverty is rampant, to increase wealth through affordable, safe housing. The organization employs three strategies to do that: creating affordable housing, designing financing models that meet the long-term needs of homeowners, and educating homeowners, renters, and policymakers about issues related to fair housing practices.

The Colonias on the Border

The region is home to the largest number of "colonias"—unincorporated communities within 150 miles of the U.S.–Mexico border—in the United States. Of the 2,000 colonias between California and Texas, more than 1,400 are in the Rio Grande Valley. About 400,000 people live in the colonias of Texas, many of them earning less than the minimum wage. Residents of colonias are among the lowest-income populations served by cdcb. Colonias typically lack basic public infrastructure, including running water, sewer, electricity, and paved roads, and the housing is seriously substandard. Located in zones where flooding is frequent, they are a haven for dengue fever and other mosquito-borne illnesses and for cholera. Sources of fresh food are scarce, fields are regularly sprayed with pesticides, access to medical care is limited, and rates of type 2 diabetes and obesity are very high for both adults and children. "When we start talking about the intentionality of poverty," said Mitchell-Bennett, "this is what it looks like up close."

Common in the area is the use of "contract for deed." A person buys a piece of property with a dollar down and a $100 monthly payment and lives in a trailer or shack on the property while the payments continue indefinitely. Contract for deed, said Mitchell-Bennett, is "a way to steal from poor people. 'I don't have to tell you how much you owe me. I don't have to disclose what you paid in principal and interest. If you miss a payment, that's mine and everything you improved on that property is mine. And oh, by the way, I told you I was going to put sewer in? Nah, I'm not going to do that.'"

Although regulation has improved the situation somewhat in recent years, there are still about 5,500 active contracts for deeds, with 450 recorded each year in 10 counties. There are also an estimated 6,500 unrecorded contracts in six counties, where an agreement may be signed but is not recorded in any city or county.

cdcb has been working in the colonias since the early 1990s, trying to improve the lives of people who just "want a piece of the American dream, to own a piece of dirt and put in their chickens and gardens," said Mitchell-Bennett. The agency is well known among low-income residents of the Rio Grande Valley, who connect with it mostly through word of mouth.

An Alternative Housing Development Model

Through its nonprofit construction company and partnerships with for-profit contractors, cdcb has built some 100 to 110 houses each year for the past five years and sold or rented them to low-income people. It also provides mortgages annually to another 40 to 50 people looking to buy an existing house.

"Choice Empowers"

The tagline "choice empowers" is fundamental to cdcb's approach to development. Before a house is built, the client meets with an architect at a partner firm to choose the details, based on their needs, preferences, and budget. One buyer might ask for a larger bathroom with two sinks, but smaller bedrooms. Another might prefer a large living room.

> *Most of our clients have never been given the choice of anything. Having been empowered by designing their own home, they become more involved in the community and better able to deal with issues that confront them.*
> —Nick Mitchell-Bennett

The rental units that cdcb builds are also unique, designed as a set of casitas (cottages) with parking spots next to each one. Conceived as a small village, a system of bioswales, which are channels used to drain rainwater, provides green space throughout the complex. The communities are very popular, both among potential renters and in the small rural markets where they are often built. "Small rural towns aren't really excited about apartment buildings," noted Mitchell-Bennett. "But 10 acres of 80 units that look like little bungalows or little farmhouses—they eat that up."

cdcb will also purchase existing apartment buildings in good locations where the owners have let the buildings deteriorate. "We are always on the hunt for properties," said Mitchell-Bennett. The goal is to keep low-income people in their homes at an affordable rate and ensure that the property is safe and sanitary, and then to rehab the units as people move out.

Financing Assistance

Ninety percent of cdcb's homeowners take out a mortgage. Using funds from equity investments, the low-income tax credit, and federal, state, and local government and private foundation grants, cdcb subsidizes buyers so they can afford housing. Rental prices are subsidized in much the same way. cdcb obtains equity or grant investments from a third party, develops new rental units or buys existing units, and uses the funding to reduce rent payments to 30% of renters' income.

Homeowner turnover is low in these communities. Residents, noted Mitchell-Bennett, "buy a house and this is the house they're going to pass on to their kids. That intergenerational transfer of wealth is extremely important. We don't lose a lot of homeowners." People rarely move, and there have been no foreclosures in 20 years. When homeowners do encounter financial trouble, cdcb works with them to restructure their mortgage as necessary.

Recently, Wells Fargo awarded cdcb a $2.5 million, 24-month grant as one of six winners of its Housing Affordability Breakthrough Challenge. cdcb is using the grant to develop its MiCASiTA program in the colonias and other areas of enduring rural poverty where high levels of subsidy are needed. The premise of MiCASiTA, Mitchell-Bennett explained, is that "we can build for a family what they can afford now." This may begin with one bedroom and bathroom, a small living area, and a food prep space. Over several years, as the owner has the resources, the home will be expanded—a new bedroom or bathroom may be added, for example: "At the end of four years, they have this completed house that they designed themselves and is the size they need, we've reduced the amount of subsidy to nothing, and we've helped them build equity from day one."

Mitchell-Bennett hopes to franchise this model in areas of persistent poverty and housing crisis around the country. cdcb is recruiting organizations to tailor the approach to local conditions as suitable, recognizing that how it looks in the Rio Grande Valley will be different from that in Appalachia, Indian Country, or the Mississippi Delta.

Sustaining Change

A package of other activities at cdcb is designed to encourage the next generation of homeowners, advocate for policy change, and strengthen communities for the future. Using its construction expertise as the foundation for a curriculum, cdcb operates YouthBuild, a school for young people, ages 16 to 24, who have dropped out of traditional school programs or been involved with the criminal justice system and now want to get their GED and job training. The Brownsville School District provides an annual grant to fund the school.

An average of 17 to 20 new students enroll annually. In less than a year, they earn their GED and also the National Center for Construction Education & Research's basic-level construction certificate. Each cohort builds one LEED-certified (an internationally recognized green building standard) house each year, and that experience is their classroom. They are paid while working on the construction site. Students can also receive certificates in manufacturing, computer building, Microsoft Office, and other skills. At the same time, they take the math, history, and English classes required for a GED. Close to 98% of graduates go on to a job or to college. "Graduation is my favorite time of the year, by far," said Mitchell-Bennett.

As another avenue toward housing equity, cdcb has launched People Policy Power, which brings policy issues to the attention of local, state, and federal elected officials through information sheets, events, blog posts, and webinars. Evictions, including how they were impacted by the pandemic, was the first issue addressed. Next up was combating the myth that housing in Brownsville is cheap. "Yes, compared to Austin incomes," Mitchell-Bennett allowed. "But if you're regular folks in Brownsville it's not. It's extremely expensive."

In still another new venture for cdcb, Mitchell-Bennett described the construction of its first majority upper-income community, a subdivision that will include 675 single-family homes and 400 rental units. Five miles of hike-and-bike trails and two parks are included, and a charter school is being built. Thirty percent of the homes in each housing phase will be sold to low-income buyers with the goal of helping them generate long-term housing equity. (The Texas pre-emption of inclusionary zoning does not apply to private developments.) Those homeowners will choose the location and model of their homes, in keeping with cdcb's commitment to choice. "It was a battle and it cost money," Mitchell-Bennett admitted, "but for us that's an equitable community."

A Final Word

As this chapter has demonstrated, the places people grow up, live, and raise their families have a huge impact on their health and life outcomes. Moreover, just where they are able to do that—and how much choice they have in the matter—often depends on their race, ethnicity, and income.

Recognizing the contributions of zoning, land use, and regulatory restrictions to ongoing inequity, some municipalities, regions, and states have begun to reconsider their approaches. A drive toward equity is also being advanced by nonprofit organizations that are assisting renters and potential homeowners to move to neighborhoods they believe will allow their families a brighter future.

Recent events have created further momentum for change. The economic impact of the pandemic and the increased attention to racial justice have finally sparked in-depth conversations about housing instability and inequitable communities in some circles. A White House memorandum issued in January 2021 acknowledged the role that the federal government has played in creating and maintaining racially discriminatory housing policies that have "contributed to segregated neighborhoods and inhibited equal opportunity and the chance to build wealth for Black, Latino, Asian American and Pacific Islander, and Native American families, and other underserved communities."[14] Substantive change is in the offing with the passage of the American Rescue Plan in March 2021, which includes nearly $50 billion to create affordable housing and provide a range of essential housing services and assistance.[15]

Indeed, turmoil may prove to have a transformative effect, broadening the movement to build more equitable housing practices and strengthen communities. As Demetria McCain noted, "It can't only be Black people, people of color, low-income people speaking up. Everybody has to speak up because this issue affects everybody. It affects all of our communities."

Spotlight

Creating a Healthy, Livable Community

Primus Wheeler, MS, Executive Director, Jackson Medical Mall Foundation

In 1970, the Jackson Mall became the first shopping mall to open in Mississippi. Initially successful, it began to deteriorate in the 1980s and was eventually abandoned by its tenants, leaving a large derelict structure as a community eyesore. In the previously thriving historical neighborhoods of Georgetown, Virden Addition, Shady Oaks, and Mid-Town where the mall is located, homeownership had dwindled to about 20% of the population, the poverty rate was over 40%, and rundown buildings were ubiquitous.

Local pediatrician Aaron Shirley, MD, would pass the old mall regularly and thought each time that something should be done with it. And so he stepped in to make that something happen, creating the Jackson Medical Mall in partnership with the University of Mississippi Medical Center, Jackson State University, and Tougaloo College. The medical mall opened its doors in 1996.

The partners agreed on a dual mission: providing healthcare for underserved populations and redeveloping the surrounding neighborhood. A community advisory board was established to ensure that the community was engaged as an equal development partner. "At the time," explained executive director Primus Wheeler, "they were thinking it had to be something very accessible to everybody in the community."

Today, the Jackson Medical Mall Foundation operates the facility, leasing space to providers and businesses who deliver most of the healthcare and ancillary services. In addition to clinics ranging from radiation/oncology to renal dialysis, offerings include a pharmacy, eye care, a childcare center, offices of Jackson State University's School of Public Health, a credit union, restaurants, and a farmers market. Some 200,000 people are served each year, mostly from

Primus Wheeler, *Spotlight* In: *Necessary Conversations*. Edited by: Alonzo L. Plough, Oxford University Press. © Robert Wood Johnson Foundation 2022. DOI: 10.1093/oso/9780197641477.003.0015

the Jackson metropolitan area, but others from across the state also seek health-care there. The goal from its inception has been to offer previously underserved clients "a very nice place to get healthcare, at appointed times, without long waits," Wheeler said.

With adjoining properties acquired through purchase or donation, the complex now covers 100 acres and employs about 1,500 people, contributing about $25 million annually in payroll to the Jackson area. The Mall Foundation has also strengthened the second pillar of its mission—community development—by building 30 new homes in the neighborhood for sale or lease-purchase (a 15-year lease followed by a 15-year mortgage). These homes are available to mall employees and others who want to live in the community. The Mall Foundation continues to purchase nearby abandoned properties and redirect them to new businesses or to affordable housing.

> *From the beginning, we wanted to reclaim the community, start to rebuild it, make it better, and create a sense of ownership so there would be a reason for folks to stay around and help keep the community strong and safe.*
> —Primus Wheeler

Now, there is a grocery store and thriving businesses that have been able to improve their storefronts. The focus remains on establishing a mix of retail and residential development as part of a long-term plan "to develop a livable community," according to Wheeler. There is still work to do, but progress is obvious: "It looks really healthy now as opposed to something that was dying on the vine," said Wheeler.

In 2015, a community assessment identified a strong interest in re-energizing local arts and culture, which had previously contributed so much to community well-being, and that become the third pillar in the mall's now-expanded mission. In 2015, ArtPlace America awarded the Mall Foundation a three-year, $3 million grant to incorporate arts and cultural programming into its work. As the organization considered how to connect healthcare, community development, and arts and culture to improve health and economic outcomes, the lack of innovation and technology in the community also became evident. A fourth pillar was put in place.

The four pillars—healthcare, community development, arts and culture, and innovation and technology—undergird the goal of preventing poor health, rather than treating it later. The Mall Foundation has rented space to artists; partnered with minority business owners to create a dance studio, media production studio, and quilting program; and launched drum corps and other programs to teach kids new skills and allow them to have fun. Science, technology, engineering, and medicine (STEM) programs are offered after school and in the summer to get young people involved in technology. The combination, as Wheeler described it, "is a multigenerational program that teaches folks how to provide for themselves."

But "teaching self-sufficiency is very difficult in this community," acknowledged Wheeler. "You have to wipe out the hopelessness first before you can get folks to start thinking 'this is something I can do for myself.'" Other programs that support this goal include a community garden, cooking classes in the mall's commercial kitchen, and a 4:30 a.m. opening that allows local residents to walk for exercise. All of the mall's programs, services, and community investments "work together to improve health and wealth outcomes," he explained.

Wheeler has great hopes for the mall's future. Plans are in the works to redesign the 50-year-old building to attract even more users. The foundation is also developing a master plan to guide the community's future and hopes to extend it to the larger Jackson community. The plan will be implemented after the pandemic subsides and may include smaller medical mall "pods" in other areas of the city. With its community partnership a key driver of development, Wheeler noted the foundation's track record with pride. "We are way ahead in redeveloping our space and creating affordable housing, new businesses, and livable communities," he said.

Transforming Research and Evaluation

Jara Dean-Coffey, MPH, Founder and Director, Equitable Evaluation Initiative; Founder and Principal, Luminare Group

Charon Gwynn, PhD, Deputy Commissioner, Division of Epidemiology, New York City Department of Health and Mental Hygiene

Donna M. Mertens, PhD, Transformative Research and Evaluation; Professor Emeritus, Gallaudet University

Alfredo Ortiz Aragón, PhD, Associate Professor, Dreeben School of Education, University of the Incarnate Word

Research can inform strategies to mitigate racism, promote social justice, and further health equity. Evaluation is a core partner in that effort, helping to measure what works and identifying opportunities to adjust and fine-tune approaches that help to achieve those broad goals. But the traditional frameworks and methodologies on which common research and evaluation practices are built can also reinforce the unjust systems that are responsible for racial and health inequities. This chapter offers perspectives on refocusing traditional research and evaluation within a rigorous, values-based framework in service to racial justice and health equity. Innovative approaches to investigation and assessment are explored as are the implications of the COVID-19 pandemic and the nation's growing racial reckoning on research and evaluation.

Jara Dean-Coffey of the Equitable Evaluation Initiative, traces the history of evaluative practice in the United States. By asking us to consider its origins and how the underlying beliefs and values limit our understanding and knowledge, she points us toward a new paradigm in which evaluation both reflects

Jara Dean-Coffey, Charon Gwynn, Donna M. Mertens, and Alfredo Ortiz Aragón, *Transforming Research and Evaluation*
In: *Necessary Conversations*. Edited by: Alonzo L. Plough, Oxford University Press. © Robert Wood Johnson Foundation
2022. DOI: 10.1093/oso/9780197641477.003.0016

and is in service of equity. At the University of the Incarnate Word, action researcher Alfredo Ortiz Aragón advocates employing the full range of ways that humans learn about the world in order to uncover new perspectives, increase the inclusion of marginalized people, and effect real social change. Gallaudet University researcher and evaluator Donna Mertens makes the case for a transformative approach to research and evaluation that captures complexity, addresses justice and equity, builds coalitions, and develops community capacity.

In the chapter's Spotlight, New York City Department of Health and Mental Hygiene epidemiologist Charon Gwynn offers an example of collaboration across institutions and between the city health department and academic researchers to develop a shared understanding of health equity and to conduct research that informs equity-directed policymaking.

Evaluation to Reflect and Serve Equity

> You don't even know me
> You say that I'm not living right
> You don't understand me
> So why do you judge my life?[1]

Jara Dean-Coffey opened her presentation at the *Sharing Knowledge* conference with a music track featuring these lyrics to emphasize that "oftentimes those who lead and use evaluative work are removed from the issue, people, place, and even politics." Power lies, she believes, in ascribing meaning to information. This power, she asserts, "drives the decisions and actions which follow and create the narrative which, over time, is believed to be truth," reinforcing a "Western-centric, White-dominant frame with strong capitalist and patriarchal undertones."

Historically, for Dean-Coffey, evaluation reflects this frame and is more often than not moored in the experiences, values, and concerns of a world that primarily privileges that which is White, heteronormative, cisgendered, and male. Evaluation is one way in which knowledge is constructed: It affirms, challenges, and may expand what we believe to be true and which narratives are seen as valid. Given the role of evaluation in the development, funding, and ongoing support of programs and initiatives that not only impact people's lives and livelihoods but also shape how we understand society and those who live within it, she believes that current frameworks upholding evaluative practice must be challenged and reimagined to create change.

The stakes are too high for evaluation to not be an instrument of change and in service of equity and liberation.

—Jara Dean-Coffey

The practice of evaluation gained prominence in the 1960s as a way to assess federal investment in social programs. Evaluation was considered to be a "practical craft,"[2] whose basic rationale was to provide "information for action,"[3] with results used to improve or terminate programs and inform decisions on policymaking. In the 1980s, professional evaluators began to work with philanthropic foundations to study the effectiveness of large programs, using the techniques, tools, and methodologies developed through federal evaluation work, which valued quantitative data and emphasized scientific rigor and validity.[4] By the 1990s, major foundations, including the Robert Wood Johnson Foundation, increased their use of evaluation to better understand the outcomes of their grantmaking.

Throughout this history, the focus of evaluation has tended to be on methodology and data from trusted sources. What this means is that the focus has been on the "how" of evaluation, with little attention to axiology (what we decide is right), ontology (what we decide is real), or epistemology (how we explore what is real and what we come to regard as fact versus opinion). By not making the underpinnings transparent and explicit, they remain uninterrogated and operate invisibly.

What if, asked Dean-Coffey, evaluations instead started with a recognition that "knowledge is socially constructed and historically located and that systems and rules must be in complex and integrated environments? What if evaluation was *for* something and embraced a myriad ways of knowing and a multiplicity of truths that coexist?"

Concentrating on Philanthropy

As founder and director of the Equitable Evaluation Initiative, Dean-Coffey works with leaders "who are reimagining the purpose and practice of evaluation to advance equity and expand notions of validity, objectivity, and rigor, and embrace complexity."[5] These leaders have been uncomfortable with traditional evaluation approaches, she said, and "think evaluative practice should be in service of a new world that centers on equity, justice, and liberation." The initiative is funded by a group of investment partners, including RWJF and other major foundations and social enterprises.

The philanthropy field is uniquely positioned to be flexible in both its allocation of resources and its decision-making. Many philanthropies have also been increasing their attention to diversity, equity, and inclusion. Thus, the five-year Equitable Evaluation Initiative, which launched in 2019 after a year of incubation, is centered on philanthropy, and particularly on foundations, which have "the greatest power within the U.S. settler-created philanthropic industrial complex," Dean-Coffey said.[6,7] The stated project goal is to seed a field of practice that embraces the complexity of evaluative work (and indeed the complexity of the world), shifting knowledge paradigms and challenging sector norms that are White-centric and exclusionary and limit what we are fully able to understand, embrace, and hold.[8]

The Equitable Evaluation Framework™

Given philanthropy's recognition that it urgently needs to understand its own knowledge paradigms, norms, and embedded biases, Dean-Coffey offers the Equitable Evaluation Framework.™ The framework seeks to examine the underpinnings of how we conceptualize knowledge, expand definitions of validity that allow for the complexity of the human experience, include those historically omitted from narratives surrounding value and truth, and challenge understandings of objectivity—bringing in multiple forms of quantitative and qualitative data and data yet conceptualized.[9] The framework is built on three principles:[10]

- **Evaluation and evaluative work should be in service of equity.** That is, the design, implementation, and use of evaluation and evaluative work must be based on a responsibility to further progress toward equity. Dean-Coffey described this first principle as "the game changer."
- **Evaluative work should be designed and implemented commensurate with the values underlying equity work.** It should be multiculturally valid and directed at participant ownership.
- **Evaluative work can and should answer critical questions** about the historical and structural decisions that have contributed to the issue under study, a strategy's effect on different groups and underlying systemic drivers of inequity, and the role of cultural context.

Building on these principles, the framework seeks to redefine six key elements of evaluation practice:[11]

- **Validity**: an expanded definition that includes the complexity of human experience
- **Rigor**: accuracy and soundness in relation to value and truth

- **Bias**: naming implicit biases in approaches and methodologies in order to make better decisions on which to use, the reasons for their use, and what to make explicit when sharing findings
- **Objectivity**: a recognition that our experience and identities shape our seeing, understanding, and believing
- **Evidence**: challenging the White-dominant frame that relies heavily on quantitative data and lacks complexity
- **Equity**: reflecting equitable principles in design and implementation.

This evolved framework for evaluation (and beyond) amplifies the voices that are woven into its fabric from original concept to eventual decision-making. Dean-Coffey paraphrases philosopher Julian Baggini to clarify the merit of this approach: "In the absence of having an objective view (God's eye view) of the universe, what is necessary to produce knowledge is the inclusion of as many perspectives as possible when creating knowledge; this variety of perspectives might then be molded into our knowledge communities." Prioritizing a multitude of perspectives discourages the dominant, socially situated perspectives that, without the multitude, otherwise gain too much authority in the production of knowledge, which ultimately produces "bad science."

A Paradigm Shift

The Equitable Evaluation Framework™ offers the potential to shift the evaluation paradigm from its traditional, White-dominant roots to one that embraces the intricacies of how humans live and interact with systems, structures, the environment, and one another. By making a case to philanthropy—a powerful funder and user of evaluation—the framework can become inculcated into practice and, in time, be increasingly viewed by foundations, practitioners, academia, and nonprofit organizations as imperative. If that goal is achieved, evaluation will be acknowledged not only as a tool for equity, but also as a field that must continuously adapt, learn, and be curious. Too, the field will remain in relationship with the use of validity, objectivity, and rigor, continuously embracing the complexity and ever-changing nature of the human experience and its limitations, oppressors, and possibilities.

The COVID-19 pandemic and the growing national attention to racial justice have brought an increased sense of urgency to the work of the Equitable Evaluation Initiative. "I've become more direct and hopefully more compelling in my case-making about who we are as a nation and what that has meant and will continue to mean unless we are different in the ways we approach this work,"

Dean-Coffey explained. The intention, she emphasized, is not to promote multiple program evaluations but to build a transformative process.

Doing community change, narrative change, systems change, or complexity is a fundamentally different endeavor.

—Jara Dean-Coffey

Leveraging Knowledge to Spur Action

Like Dean-Coffey, Alfredo Ortiz Aragón is motivated by a desire for a fundamentally different way to gather and use knowledge to contribute to meaningful social change. His embrace of action research began in international development work in Africa and Latin America, where he found himself reaching for "creative methodologies" to engage local people's knowledge. But even when the work went well, he felt that he and his team were not always digging deep enough: "We were being creative yet superficial, failing to leverage knowledge that was deeply relevant to people's lives."

Ortiz Aragón also noticed times when "a deep conversation would emerge—something emotional or powerful—that allowed people to see themselves in relation to one another and see their organization differently." But the capacity-building (similar to organizational development) approaches he and his colleagues used were not planned to accommodate this and the team did not adapt its approach. "Just as the conversations were finally getting to really important things," he said, "we would tie everything up in a bow in an action plan and the learning would cease. This could not have been the purpose of change processes—to cut off conversation and learning."

Committed to staying in the field of international development but going in a new direction, Ortiz Aragón completed a doctoral program at the Institute of Development Studies in Brighton, U.K. His orientation to capacity building changed from developing strategies or initiatives as an outsider to coming to an understanding of "how we as practitioners and researchers are actually part of the broader systems we engage in and can effect change at a very local level if we can get to meaningful conversations."

Methodology, Ortiz Aragón realized, was not neutral. "Even methods that we think are neutral, in fact, have a status quo worldview behind them, which will tend to favor the most powerful in a situation," he said. Therefore, he sought to rethink his approach so that his methods would respond to the people they were meant to help. He realized that could happen only if local people were actively involved in the work, in some cases to the extent of co-designing the project and methodology.

You can't engage in real transformative work if you're doing everything for someone else.

—Alfredo Ortiz Aragón

One example is a process that Ortiz Aragón and his colleague Raphael Hoetmer, regional advisor for strategy and impact in the Americas at Amnesty International, conducted in the southern highlands of Peru.[12] Their goal was to reinforce the participation of local communities and organizations in planning, decision-making, and evaluating a regional strategy for a human rights and rural development program.

The reasons to support local participation are threefold: ethical (people have a right to participate in decisions that affect them), practical (if people's voices are not heard and respected, they are unlikely to buy in to the resulting actions), and strategic (people closest to the issues possess the fundamental knowledge needed for the process to succeed). "If the people aren't involved, who is this for?" he asked. Ortiz Aragón and the other project facilitators employed a range of reflective methods, including drawings, shared timelines, and mapping to foster engagement.

At one point in the process, when discussion about painful or uncomfortable topics seemed to stall, the facilitators turned to skits. Women who had been very quiet up to that point suddenly opened up as they acted out scenes of rural violence directed at women. Without facilitator prompting, participants conducted more than half of the skits in their native Quechua, rather than Spanish. This was a lightbulb moment for the foreign facilitators. "Why didn't we think of that?" they wondered. "Why did we assume that this entire process could be legitimately done in Spanish just because we were in Peru?" After much reflection, not only about their use of language but also about their assumptions that presentations and discussions were the right tools, Ortiz Aragón and Hoetmer acknowledged, "Our eyes were opened to how little we were paying attention to how people actually live and share their knowledge with each other."

Action Research Fundamentals

From that insight, Ortiz Aragón further committed to action research, which is built on three key ideas: participation by those who know (those closest to the issues who know the most), acting to learn (taking action to generate knowledge), and learning to act (harvesting knowledge from action).[13]

Participation by Those Who Know

People closest to the ground have the most relevant knowledge to share, making their participation in the research process especially important. And while humans come to know the world in multiple ways, research tools are typically limited to observation, focus groups, interviews, and surveys. "We can get true participation by asking people to tell us how they learn and by breaking out of narrow ways of seeing the world methodologically," Ortiz Aragón stressed. Traditional research methods can indeed generate knowledge that leads to improvement and change, but so too can integration of social media, performance, informal conversation, and the many other ways in which people gather information and knowledge.

In order to fully include the knowledge-holders—people who are living the situation under study—in the research, it is not enough just to invite them in. Rather, they must also be able to shape the actions that emerge. Whether they are park rangers in Ecuador or LGBTQ+ community members in San Antonio, community actors must have influence and researchers must be willing and able to adapt previously developed plans to follow their direction. Ortiz Aragón called this the most important component of truly inclusive action research.

Acting to Learn

A core component of "acting to learn" is taking action with the intention to contribute to some sort of change or improvement. An example is Action Research in Support of Community Health and Wellbeing, a partnership he and his research team at the University of the Incarnate Word in San Antonio, Texas, have forged with the city's Healthy Neighborhoods Program, with funding from RWJF.[14] Through this program, students and faculty, community health workers, and community actors seek to do three things:

- **Increase participation of community actors in their own health and well-being.** Two examples: contributing toward more equitable access to and treatment of LGBTQ+ people in healthcare settings and helping increase access to services for children with autism by working with their parents (as described below). This requires inviting community knowledge-holders, creating spaces for sharing, using methods that allow for sharing, and co-designing and co-facilitating strategies for action.
- **Intentionally document knowledge.** Examples include creating digital stories, data visuals, presentations, and reports that gather and analyze insights from interviews and focus groups. This requires highlighting and valuing the community knowledge that emerges, paying attention to and mapping problems and potential solutions that are found within stories, making knowledge visible and understandable through visualized data, and becoming reflective practitioners.
- **Use that documented knowledge to inform action.** Examples include engaging in community conversations; doing presentations; developing

educational materials; advocating, organizing, and networking; and taking small actions. This requires documenting and processing knowledge in agile and usable forms, mapping opportunities for influence, testing out actions for their learning and influence potential, and moving from thinking to acting, reflecting, and evaluating.

Fundamental to this process, noted Ortiz Aragón, is the collaboration that envelops the entirety of the effort. Those involved have a multitude of titles and positions (practitioner, community health worker, professor, nurse, supervisor, physical therapist, action researcher, student, community member) and also bring unique experiences that "provide opportunities that both enable and constrain our important work together," he said. The work is also enabled and constrained, he continued, "by the cultural and power relationships that are prevalent in the institutions to which we belong."

This commitment to collaboration requires "creating mechanisms and opportunities to negotiate power and to learn one another's lingo, strengths and weaknesses, communication styles, and identities, and to create 'team' when it makes sense," Ortiz Aragón observed. The key, he said, is to make an effort to find complementarities and opportunities to become stronger together in a ways that allow them to become more than the sum of their parts.

Importantly, action research elevates this relationship-building. "To what extent will the process we have used generate goodwill, empathetic relationships, ethical processes, momentum, synergies, and a desire to keep working together?" asked Ortiz Aragón. This is a central question, he explained, because a strong relationship base can support the readiness and willingness to act into the future and build the networks that make that possible. Moreover, as "we invest in really getting to know each other and create opportunities for each of us to participate, do our best work, and hear and be heard in shared language that makes sense to everyone, we increase our chances of being relevant to the causes we aim to support."

Acting to learn also includes going beyond reading, observing, and gathering information to take small actions that open up a world of learning about how others experience their lives. These might include engaging in conversation, attending an event, or taking an elderly person to buy groceries as a way to understand social isolation more directly.[15] In each case, by engaging more personally with people, the researcher becomes a participant in the process as well as an observer.

Learning to Act

Practitioners are always "acting," Ortiz Aragón contends. They are busy getting things done. But they tend not to be trained to slow down, reflect, harvest knowledge, and leverage that knowledge to inform action. It is important, he stressed, to find ways to increase reflective practice so that their learning can be available to inform action. In training researchers, Ortiz Aragón espouses a hybrid between the "ungrounded academic" who is always "in the clouds" and far from action and the "unthinking practitioner" who is always "doing" but not leveraging the available knowledge to bring purpose to the doing. The goal of the hybrid approach is better, more thoughtful reflective action.[16]

Employing Action Research to Advance Equity

Several examples illustrate how an action research approach can support gains in health equity. In an example of acting to learn, the team built on findings from a previous focus group and connected members of the LGBTQ+ community with a class of 50 pre-health profession students in several gatherings. After LGBTQ+ participants told stories of poor treatment at the hands of the healthcare system, the group reflected on those stories and then the storytellers retold them as they wished they had unfolded—"rewriting the script" in the process. As part of the project, the students created visuals designed to educate and influence others, used the visuals in other settings (such as with family or friends, or even in clinical settings during an internship), and shared back their experiences with the LGBTQ+ community members. "This emergent process allows us to generate knowledge from experience and use that knowledge to think of new ways to continue the inquiries that could influence change," said Ortiz Aragón.

In another example, parents and caretakers of children on the autism spectrum shared their stories about accessing services. They then created and presented digital stories to help them feel heard, connected, and motivated to improve access in the future. Over time, the parents and researchers will determine how best to use these stories to build awareness of their experiences in the hope of furthering more equitable treatment.

In each of these cases, and in action research in general, the aim is not just to get the stories out, Ortiz Aragón explained, but to use them to help people connect the dots and figure out how they can have influence and generate change strategies.

> *Inviting people to participate in action and reflective research processes can yield tangible improvements and contribute to addressing racial injustice, human rights, and improved health outcomes. When we ask "who knows" and how they know, we can put that into cycles of action and reflection.*
> —Alfredo Ortiz Aragón

A Transformative Approach to Research and Evaluation

The desire to further social justice and improve people's lives also motivated Donna Mertens as she developed her transformative approach to research and evaluation. The seed for her aspiration was planted when she was growing up in Kentucky in the early 1960s. In that innocent way of children, she was perplexed by the conditions in which her Black peers lived, which were so vastly different from her own. She recalled a nagging awareness that something was wrong and wanted to understand more about the causes and how they could be changed.

Learning of the Civil Rights Movement, she wondered whether it had made a difference. Raising what she called "an evaluative question" opened her eyes to the power of research and evaluation—a personally "transformative moment" that began to frame her approach to understanding social justice and how to mitigate it.

As a young professional, Mertens collected data about the need for continuing education for the Appalachian Regional Commission and later gathered vocational education data. Although she felt a strong need to spend time with people impacted by the programs she was studying, rather than confining her analyses to national surveys, that wasn't part of her assignment. The lack of "the immersion experience of being connected, in a meaningful way, with a population that experiences marginalization" became acutely frustrating to her.

Mertens eventually found the experience she sought in a position teaching research and evaluation at Gallaudet University in Washington, the only university in the world that serves deaf students through direct communication using American Sign Language. Until then, Mertens knew nothing about deaf culture nor could she communicate because she did not know sign language. Indeed, she had never even met someone who could not hear. The deaf students provided the transformative opportunities she needed to understand better how to conduct research and evaluation that could lead to increased justice for this community.

But she learned quickly, becoming as much student as educator herself. Her students described being excluded from research and evaluation, telling her, "Conclusions are drawn that make us look bad, because people don't understand our language and our culture. And most of the research is done by hearing people." Mertens drew on feminist literature about discrimination, oppression, and lived experience as a guide to thinking about research and evaluation. "Just change 'woman' to 'deaf' and you've got it," agreed her students.

With their encouragement, Mertens began to develop methodologies that recognized the heterogeneity and intersectionality within the deaf community. "Deaf people represent a microcosm of society," she said. "They come in all colors, genders, sexual identities, and from different countries and economic classes." She soon realized the same approach to research could be broadly applied to other marginalized populations.

Transformative work, stressed Mertens, means not working from assumptions about the problem and its solution. Nor is it looking at evaluation only as a way to determine program effectiveness. Rather, it means doing a great deal of upfront work to define the problem being addressed and consider whose voice has been privileged in understanding that problem.

Engaging Community Voices

The transformative approach uses many typical data collection methods, such as surveys, interviews, and focus groups when they are appropriate. What makes it distinctive, said Mertens, is that it begins by asking who should be engaged in the work and how that should happen:[17] "Whose voices are coming into the early understanding of what it is that we're trying to focus on? And, if there are missing voices, what strategies are needed to invite those voices in ways that aren't just tokenism, but are supportive and which provide safe space, because in some contexts people may lose their job or not get needed services if their voices are heard."

Determining how best to involve people closest to the issue "is very contextually determined," said Mertens. The literature can provide a starting point, but inclusion in the literature is a position of privilege, one that is often unavailable to the people most affected. Mertens recommends reaching out to community groups, grassroots organizations, and churches to find trusted community members who are already engaged in the work and asking them for advice on connecting with others. "It's coming in with an attitude of humility," she advised.

Once involved, those community members can be asked about the best ways to collect data and the questions they believe to be most relevant. Strategies for working together are needed so that when differing viewpoints surface, the voices of those who are traditionally powerful don't dominate. The goal, according to Mertens, is to use available research tools to make sure that this "really suits where we are working and what we need to know." Coalitions can also help ensure that the community has the data it needs to sustain the work after a formal evaluation ends. Using a collaborative approach from the outset lays the groundwork for sustainability. Throughout, relationship-building and contextual analysis are key, even for a pilot study, Mertens said, so that the study is responsive to "the cultural context and the complexity where you are working."

> *Respectful engagement with stakeholders—with an intention to address problems within a context of understanding historically, legislatively, economically, and politically why people are experiencing the things they're experiencing—leads us to develop interventions with potentially greater impact than doing something that we just think is right.*
>
> —Donna Mertens

The early response from the field to Mertens's ideas was skeptical at best, but today, "especially with the prevalence of sustainable development goals throughout the global community, 'transformation' is everywhere," she said. "I am heartened that is now a word in common parlance and that people see it as an appropriate goal for the work we do."

Theoretical Underpinnings and Methodological Choices

Mertens pointed to the increased use of systems theory and complexity theory to support the importance of analyzing the larger context in which a problem exists. Such analysis is especially important when the goal is systems change because understanding the historical experience of marginalized people is critical for transformation. An example is recognizing the connection between a neighborhood's racial composition and the likelihood of nearby toxic waste dumps, and how that inequity originated in the discriminatory practices that are part of the history of the United States (see Chapter 7 for a fuller description of "dumping" on people of color).

Like Ortiz Aragón, Mertens is a strong advocate of mixed-methods research, which can include traditional surveys and focus groups but also skits, artwork, conversation, and poetry—whatever people are most comfortable using to share information. The combination of quantitative and qualitative data can be powerful, but she pointed out that qualitative methods don't necessarily have to involve words.

A transformative approach can also be integrated into more traditionally designed research or evaluation projects, providing a mechanism for community input and enriching the potential for enhanced outcomes. To evaluate an HIV/AIDS prevention education program, for example, her team worked with two advisory groups—one community-based, the other youth-based—to design an intervention that the youth felt would work for them, and then conducted a randomized controlled trial on that intervention.

Hope for the Future

The renewed focus on racial justice in 2020 brought greater attention to the structure of evaluations. Mertens believes that it has also highlighted the importance of evaluators working closely with grassroots organizations, adopting the strategies of social activists, and expanding their approach to injustice, poverty, and health disparities. The COVID-19 pandemic, too, has raised awareness of inequity, helping to make the time right for a transformative approach to evaluation. Mertens is hopeful that more opportunities will emerge, citing two examples that represent the evolution of the field:

- Her team worked with Engineers Without Borders to develop a toolkit[18] and author a chapter in an impact investing handbook[19] to support the use of social impact investing as a contribution to social justice.
- Mertens and her colleague, Bagele Chilisa, PhD, at the University of Botswana, addressed the lack of Indigenous approaches and voices in evaluation in an *American Journal of Evaluation* article.[20] "Indigenous people have their own worldviews," stressed Merton, arguing that Western-dominant evaluation approaches do not adequately recognize and incorporate the culture, ethics, and values of Indigenous perspectives and paradigms.

In the future, I would like to see this transformative lens being brought into contexts where it hasn't been before to address social, economic, and environmental justice.

—Donna Mertens

A Final Word

As the contributors to this chapter make clear, research and evaluation practices and outcomes have a significant impact on how racial injustice and health inequity are defined, discussed, and addressed. Traditional Western-centric and White-dominant frames have dictated much of the history of research and evaluation practice, limiting the innovations that might be used to tackle longstanding issues of racism, poverty, and health inequities.

The values-based approaches offered here are united in emphasizing the need to deeply engage the people confronting the problem under study; the importance of understanding context and complexity when seeking system change; and the willingness to employ the full range of methods that people use to share knowledge, from long-established methodologies to more unconventional information-gathering strategies. They also share the common goal of reorienting research and evaluation practice in transformative and even radical ways in pursuit of equity, justice, and social change while remaining committed to rigor—indeed, rigor is advanced and strengthened through this transformation. A recharged emphasis on the health and social impacts of structural racism only adds to the urgency.

Spotlight

Racial Equity and Social Justice in City Health Department Practices

Charon Gwynn, PhD, Deputy Commissioner, Division of Epidemiology, New York City Department of Health and Mental Hygiene

The New York City Department of Health and Mental Hygiene is one of the largest health departments in the world, with over 6,000 public health practitioners, according to Deputy Commissioner Charon Gwynn. Although the department's stated goal is to promote and protect the health of all New Yorkers, it is part of a broader system whose discriminatory institutional practices have contributed to long-standing health disparities in the city. Two initiatives were designed to confront that reality.

In 2015, then Health Commissioner Mary T. Bassett, MD, MPH, created the Race to Justice Initiative to "examine all of our policies and practices internally to ensure that race equity and social justice are reflected in everything that we do," said Gwynn. She explained that Bassett was explicit about shifting the department's focus from disparity as a socioeconomic issue to identifying it as a racial equity issue that reflected historical disinvestment and structural racism: "Her thinking was to first name that and then, as an institution, recognize how our own systems contribute to that."

The Race to Justice Initiative is now a permanent part of the agency under the direction of a chief equity officer. The ongoing goal of the initiative is to develop and implement policies and practices that take aim at health disparities. One notable accomplishment is the development of the Race to Justice Action Kit, which offers resources for use across the department to strengthen

Charon Gwynn, *Spotlight* In: *Necessary Conversations*. Edited by: Alonzo L. Plough, Oxford University Press. © Robert Wood Johnson Foundation 2022. DOI: 10.1093/oso/9780197641477.003.0017

its communications and community engagement and align it with racial equity and social justice practices.

In March 2019, the department launched a pilot initiative, Health Data for New York City or HD4NYC, in partnership with the New York Academy of Medicine and with funding from the Robert Wood Johnson Foundation, to enhance the use of department data to promote health equity.[1] As the Race to Justice Initiative strives to identify and reduce health disparities, collecting and analyzing health data—essential activities at any health department to inform policy and programming—are critical. Department data sources include birth and death records, telephone and in-person surveys, hospital discharges, and disease registries that are available to researchers from both the health department and academic institutions. But each group faces limitations: The department's applied researchers may lack the resources or time to use innovative research methods, while academic researchers may be unfamiliar with the data and health department priorities and lack access to department datasets.

The three-year HD4NYC initiative aims to address these barriers. The objective is to build collaboration across institutions and between the department's applied researchers and academic researchers in order "to cultivate the next generation of public health researchers with a commitment to health equity" who can produce policy-relevant research that can reduce health disparities, said Gwynn.

> *Data is a key part of the way that we advance health equity in New York City. Leveraging public–private partnerships can be a win-win.*
> —Charon Gwynn

Initiative participation was competitive, ultimately bringing together eight applied researchers from five health department divisions and 17 academic investigators from 13 New York City institutions and reflects a cross-section of disciplines and interests.

HD4NYC fosters an infrastructure to facilitate collaboration and expand data use through a working group model and mentorship from established agency and academic researchers. In line with health department priorities, two working groups have been formed: One focuses on marginalized populations, the other on birth and childhood equity. After a series of group discussions and a review of data sources, the groups identified research questions in six areas:

- Health and economic impacts of banning menthol cigarettes
- Police contacts and health
- Bullying among LGBTQ youth of color

- Maternal healthcare among immigrants
- Health of children in immigrant families
- Children's environmental health

Participating in HD4NYC brings professional benefits to both groups of researchers. Applied health department researchers are exposed to the innovative tools, methodologies, and analyses used in academic research while academic researchers learn how to access health department datasets and gain insights into the department's programmatic interests. The professional working relationships forged through this work can also lead to future collaborations, with a goal of facilitating deep and meaningful engagement of stakeholders throughout the research process. Moreover, at a systems level, these partnerships expand and strengthen health equity research and the potential for policy and program changes that reduce health disparities and promote equity.

A forthcoming special section of the *Journal of Urban Health* will present papers outlining the research that emerged from the two working groups. In the future, Gwynn hopes "to find ways to have these groups help answer some of our priority questions while we're wading through the pandemic and the public health crisis of racism."

> *Our hope is that this initiative will result in longstanding collaborations, that applied and academic researchers will have a shared understanding of health equity, and that together we can conduct impactful research that informs policies and ultimately reduces health disparities.*
>
> —Charon Gwynn

Racial Justice Through Civic Engagement

A Look at Voting and the Census

Iyanrick John, JD, MPH, Adjunct Professor, California State University, East Bay

Sean Morales-Doyle, JD, Deputy Director, Voting Rights & Elections, Brennan Center for Justice at New York University School of Law

Jamal R. Watkins, Senior Vice President for Strategy and Advancement, NAACP

Civic engagement is a cornerstone of American life, linking individuals to their communities, community concerns to equitable policies, and policies to the promotion of a stable and trusted democracy. When people cast a vote, participate in a neighborhood clean-up effort, join a protest march, or run for office, they are working to shape the society in which they live, whether locally, regionally, or nationally. Civic engagement holds the potential of promoting justice and giving people faith that their voices are heard, but as earlier chapters in this book have demonstrated, not all voices have been welcome.

This chapter examines two foundational forms of civic engagement, voting and census participation. Together, election outcomes and census counts determine who leads the country; who holds power at the local, state, and national levels; who gets to establish policy; and who receives its benefits. Historically, voting and the census have been used both as tools for advancing racial justice and equity and as weapons to impede them.

The contributors—a long-time activist, an attorney, and a health policy analyst—turn their attention to civic engagement in an era of political discord, racial injustice, and a devastating pandemic. The 2020 election and census

Iyanrick John, Sean Morales-Doyle, and Jamal R. Watkins, *Racial Justice Through Civic Engagement* In: *Necessary Conversations*. Edited by: Alonzo L. Plough, Oxford University Press. © Robert Wood Johnson Foundation 2022.
DOI: 10.1093/oso/9780197641477.003.0018

count landed in the midst of a divisive political climate marked by anger, mistrust, and misinformation designed to confuse people about voting rules and frighten them about the use of census data. Both resulted in cases before the U.S. Supreme Court, and anger over the election outcome devolved into the January 6, 2021, armed assault on the U.S. Capitol. The health and economic strains of COVID-19 heightened the tensions. The virus precluded in-person, get-out-the-vote and get-out-the-census activism, while piling enormous administrative challenges on overburdened officials and advocates who lacked resources to address them.

Jamal Watkins opens the chapter, using the lens of the NAACP's long history and wide reach to reflect broadly on the nature of civic engagement. Then, Sean Morales-Doyle of the Brennan Center for Justice at New York University School of Law explores tools of voter suppression, their use through the 2020 election cycle, and the implications going forward. The chapter concludes with insights from the Asian & Pacific Islander American Health Forum's Iyanrick John about the role of the census in promoting democracy and the challenges in ensuring full participation, using Asian Americans, Native Hawaiians, and Pacific Islanders as examples.

Pragmatic Tools for Progress and Innovation

Jamal Watkins, senior vice president for strategy and advancement at the NAACP, wants the organization and its constituents to "wake up with progress and innovation on our minds in working to overcome whatever barriers we face." He uses a pragmatic, community-driven action agenda to strive toward that progress.

As a large organization with both national and local agendas, the NAACP reaches deep into communities, propelled by the work of more than half a million members, 2,200 branch or unit offices, and 2 million volunteers.[1] It has honed a strategy in which shared national or regional priorities frame and support local activities. Civic engagement, Watkins believes, happens when individuals participate in policy development and implementation processes that directly affect their own well-being and that of their communities. "Civic engagement is the tool, but policy solutions are the destination," he said.

Recognizing that the Black community is not a monolith, Watkins emphasizes the importance of research to identify issues of most importance to local residents. Economic stability and healthcare emerge as two widely shared concerns, he said, while noting that the kinds of jobs offering economic stability and the forms of healthcare delivery yielding the best outcomes will differ significantly across communities.

The wins are tailored to communities, but there are universal threads.
—Jamal Watkins

The NAACP's priorities since its inception in 1909 have been eliminating racial disparities and promoting inclusion of people whose voices often go unheard, according to Watkins. In considering whether the NAACP should pursue an initiative, he asks, "If this particular policy doesn't impact racial disparities and if it isn't linked to being inclusive, does it fit with what we should be prioritizing?"

Watkins described three core NAACP civic engagement strategies:

- Driving Black turnout for elections, both to register eligible voters and then to ensure that registered voters turn out on Election Day.
- Developing civic leaders. The organization's membership and volunteer network are designed to build community leadership capable of engaging residents to advocate for themselves and their communities. "We are about volunteers engaging and leading in a hyper-local way," Watkins explained.
- Educating its members and the general public on the connection between civic engagement, equitable policies, and democracy. Convincing people of the importance of the census requires education, for example, since "redistricting is not often a dinner-table conversation," Watkins acknowledged with a chuckle.

Civic Engagement in a Pandemic

The pandemic has unveiled both cracks and strengths in the nation's capacity for civic engagement. In some incidents, people have acted on their own by refusing vaccinations or protective face coverings or by gathering in large indoor groups, insisting that doing so is a matter of personal freedom. In others, neighbors have engaged with one another for the first time, organizing free clothing and food distribution systems or purchasing meals in bulk from struggling neighborhood restaurants to be delivered to essential workers.

These kinds of actions demonstrate the connection between civic engagement and public health policies, Watkins said. Protests by healthcare workers and teachers over inadequate health and safety protocols have led to policy and system-wide standards for ventilation, cleaning, and the use of personal protection equipment, for example. RWJF's Culture of Health has been helpful to the NAACP, Watkins noted, by offering a way for both activists and policymakers to frame good health as more than receiving good clinical care.

How do we engage people in leveraging the COVID-19 crisis for the public good?

—Jamal Watkins

Technology is one area ripe for leveraging. The pressures of COVID-19 prompted families, nonprofit organizations, school officials, and businesses to advocate for structural improvements in home internet access. These improvements, which are likely to continue as the pandemic wanes, have implications for access to education, economic opportunity, and full participation in many other dimensions of society. "Technology limitations that were perceived as annoying in the past became life changing," Watkins explained.

COVID-19 also prompted the NAACP to become more creative with its own in-house technical capacity, broadening the reach of its civic engagement agenda. "We had to switch to Zoom events," Watkins said, describing the NAACP's departure from its long history of on-the-ground activism. That required significant adjustments, but it also came with benefits: "I can participate in a Zoom event with 15 cities rather than go in person to just a few cities."

Voting, Racial Justice, and Health Equity

Sean Morales-Doyle's commitment to legal and policy work at New York University's Brennan Center for Justice grew out of childhood experiences attending community meetings and protest marches with his activist parents. "Voting was a family priority, but I learned from my parents a more expansive view of what civic engagement was like," he said. "It is an opportunity to intertwine policy work with community work."

Watching his father mobilize residents to advocate for a stop sign at a dangerous intersection taught Morales-Doyle an early lesson about the value of small wins. "This isn't the ultimate fight," he recalls his father explaining, "but you do this first because people see they can win, and that gives them agency."

To ensure that agency, institutions have to encourage people to engage, and then respect their perspectives when they do. "Efforts to prevent people from expressing their beliefs send a powerful, damaging message to them about the significance of their voices and their ability to effect change," Morales-Doyle said, adding, "Democracy doesn't work if people don't believe in it."

There are many ways to undermine that belief, beginning with interfering in the most fundamental tool of a democracy: the right to vote.

The Three Prongs of Voter Suppression

Exclusionary voting practices have a long history in the United States, well matched by an equally long history of determined efforts to broaden the franchise. These are best understood by examining three long-standing voter suppression tactics: disenfranchisement, barriers, and misinformation.

Disenfranchisement

In this most obvious suppression strategy, certain groups have been legally barred from voting. From the ratification of the Constitution in 1790 until the 15th Amendment was ratified in 1870, only White men were usually allowed to vote. The 15th Amendment ostensibly extended voting rights to all men, but state laws and practices effectively rescinded those rights for many Black people.[2,3]

The 19th Amendment, ratified in 1920, gave women the right to vote,[4] although it did not remove the restrictive practices states used to circumvent the 15th Amendment, keeping many Black women ineligible.[5] Native Americans were only deemed to be U.S. citizens with passage of the Snyder Act in 1924,[6] and so were ineligible to vote until that year. Similarly, Chinese American immigrants were not permitted to apply for citizenship and therefore not allowed to vote, until 1943, when naturalization rules began to change.[7]

Disenfranchisement today takes the form of many state laws limiting people with felony convictions from voting, a policy often rooted in Civil War–era efforts to circumvent the 15th Amendment. (See Chapter 5 for a broader discussion of incarceration.)

The policy continues to disproportionally disenfranchise Black people. An October 2020 analysis from The Sentencing Project reported that more than 5.1 million people are forbidden to vote because of felony convictions, including 2.23 million who have completed their sentences. The report documented that Black people are 3.7 times more likely to be disenfranchised than non-Black people.[8]

While state disenfranchisement policies vary, the trend has been toward reinstating rights. "No states now permanently disenfranchise all people convicted of a felony, though some still permanently disenfranchise people with convictions of some, but not all felony crimes," said Morales-Doyle. Only Maine, Vermont, and Washington, D.C., however, allow all people with felony convictions to vote, including while incarcerated; 20 other states restore voting rights upon release from prison.[9] Between 2018 and 2021, 12 states and Washington, D.C., used a variety of methods, including citizen-led referenda, constitutional amendments, executive orders, and legislation, to restore some voting rights to this group.[10]

Barriers

Barriers "stop people from voting who everyone agrees are allowed to vote and to whom the laws clearly give the right to vote," Morales-Doyle explained. Typically presented as race-neutral attempts to protect against alleged voter fraud, these barriers inevitably make voting especially difficult in communities of color and low-income communities.

Civil rights laws of the 1950s and early 1960s expanded voting rights but were not adequate to remove barriers in many states.[11] Only with passage of the landmark Voting Rights Act of 1965, which prohibited barriers such as literacy tests and poll taxes, did disparities between Black and White voter registration significantly decrease.

But other obstacles remain, including onerous identification requirements, arbitrary and restrictive registration protocols, and inadequate numbers of polling places. The claim that these will prevent fraud, said Morales-Doyle, is "a false rhetoric that may make intuitive sense, but isn't true. These barriers appeal to people's fears about groups they perceive as 'others' who are coming to take something away from them."

Recent years have witnessed alarming curtailment of voting rights in some states and through U.S. Supreme Court rulings that supported their policies. In 2013, the court decision in *Shelby County [Alabama] v. Holder* rendered inoperable a key provision of the Voting Rights Act, which had required jurisdictions with histories of racial discrimination to obtain federal clearance before changing their election rules. In a 5–4 decision, the court ruled that the formula used to identify the jurisdictions subject to preclearance was out of date, essentially eliminating the preclearance system[12] and considerably reducing the law's impact.

Then, during the 2020 presidential election, litigation came to the fore as a tactic to curtail voting, with the president and his allies filing 62 election-related lawsuits in state and federal courts to inhibit vote-counting.[13] Many of them took direct aim at Black and low-income communities and voters, including in predominately Black areas of Detroit, Philadelphia, and other cities. These were "pretty thinly veiled appeals to people's xenophobia and racism," said Morales-Doyle.

The lawsuits prevailed only once, in a Pennsylvania ruling that affected few votes and did not change the outcome in the state. Nonetheless, the climate of intimidation established by the threat of litigation may have dissuaded some people from voting in the first place.

The emergence of COVID-19 upended the 2020 voting environment with a push–pull effect—additional barriers were erected, purportedly in the name of safety, but opportunities to vote early or by mail were expanded to curb infections.

> *There was a big battle over whether we were going to make it hard or easy for people to cast their votes in a healthy way during the pandemic.*
>
> —Sean Morales-Doyle

The pandemic bombarded public officials with obstacles to operating a fair election. Unprecedented numbers of mail-in and early ballots had to be collected, secured, and counted. Breakdowns in the U.S. Postal Service jeopardized the timely submission of mail-in ballots. CDC-compliant health and safety protocols required changes in polling station design and costly expenditures on personal protective equipment. These burdens fell most heavily on state and local officials who often lacked staff, space, funds, technology, and security systems to address them. Nonetheless, Christopher Krebs, the nation's most senior cybersecurity official, called the election "the most secure in American history."[14]

Looking back at the election, Morales-Doyle commented, "This was a year that connected democracy and health. I have thought far more about how voting itself is impacted by public health." In August 2020, the Brennan Center for Justice and the Infectious Diseases Society of America issued joint guidelines for in-person voting during the pandemic.

Meanwhile, the struggle over voting rights continues. The most recent twist came in July 2021 with a Supreme Court decision in *Brnovich v. Democratic National Committee*. By a 6–3 vote, the court ruled in favor of two Arizona policies that lower courts had found to be racially discriminatory: One required election officials to discard ballots cast at the wrong precinct (even ballots for national or statewide candidates), and the other barred anyone other than a family member or caregiver from returning early ballots for another person.[15]

Emboldened by the Supreme Court ruling, Texas proposed its own set of restrictive voting laws. On May 30, 2021, and again on July 12, House Democrats walked out of the legislative session devoted to the new rules in order to prevent the quorum required for a vote. Those efforts forestalled action for some time, but the legislation passed in August 2021 and Governor Greg Abbott signed it into law on September 7, 2021.[16]

Misinformation

Misinformation sows mistrust about voting by steering people to the wrong polling place, misleading them about the hours of voting, confusing them about the process, and other such tactics, explained Morales-Doyle.

One of the ways to suppress the vote is to make people not believe in it.
—Sean Morales-Doyle

Misinformation during the 2020 election featured allegations that votes were being cast illegally, voting machines were malfunctioning, and election workers were inept or corrupt. Much misinformation was aimed at Black and low-income areas. For example, these allegations were reported on National Public Radio:[17]

"Robocalls that went to tens of thousands of minority voters in Michigan, Pennsylvania, Ohio, Illinois, and New York . . . falsely claimed that voting by mail could be dangerous."

"President Trump . . . repeatedly claimed that [mail-in] ballots were abandoned in a ditch in Wisconsin, although that is not true."

"Facebook posts have warned voters that their ballot will be invalidated if a poll worker puts a mark on it, including their initials, even though that's a requirement in many states."

In response, civil rights organizations and election officials of both parties launched public information campaigns to set the record straight, offering extensive details about traditionally arcane ballot processing protocols in order to demonstrate the layers of protection and security built into the electoral system. "Election officials, no matter what their party, believe their job is to run a good election, and if they did that and are accused of not doing that, they will speak out," emphasized Morales-Doyle.

Encouraging Indications and Reasons for Concern

The 2020 election became a battle between those working to promote expansive and transparent processes and those determined to shrink, cloud, or dismantle them, strategies that culminated in an armed insurrection in the halls of Congress. The country emerged with its democratic institutions generally intact, albeit noticeably frayed and fragile.

By the time the election approached, most people did have a more accurate understanding and realistic expectations about how the outcomes would be determined, Morales-Doyle believes. "Polling showed that most people did not expect to receive election results immediately, and that was really important," he said. "The string of wins in lawsuits also helped give people confidence."

Yet deep and disturbing divides remain, and many people still justify efforts to set aside votes in Black communities, said Morales-Doyle: "That belief and other events reveal how much of our country is comfortable with fairly explicit racism."

The January 6, 2021, assault by an overwhelmingly White mob refusing to accept the election results was met with a law enforcement response that differed starkly from the much more militarized one used against peaceful marches by Black Lives Matter and other peaceful protestors. "What we saw today is a clear demonstration that many White people would rather live in a White dictatorship than in a multiracial democracy," observed a writer in *America: The Jesuit Review*.[18]

Looking ahead, there are reasons for continued concern over voter suppression as well as opportunities to reduce it. Jamal Watkins noted that the NAACP sees greatest engagement among its constituents during election seasons. "We have to leverage those moments," he stressed, because people tend to turn to other issues when an election is over." The NAACP's civic engagement activities through the U.S. Senate runoff election in Georgia helped drive turnout, and Watkins plans to build on that momentum: "The election created an opportunity, and we applied the mechanics to drive voter engagement. Now, we need those same voters to hold officials accountable."

Clearly, that work needs to be done. A July 2021 post[19] from the Brennan Center for Justice reported that between January 1 and July 14, 2021, at least 18 states enacted 30 laws that restrict voting access, and 61 restrictive bills were pending in state legislatures. Particularly draconian legislation was signed into law in Florida, Georgia, and Texas. At the same time, at least 25 states enacted 54 laws expanding voting access, including in Massachusetts, New Jersey, and Virginia. "There is reason to be worried, but we can't let our worry get the best of us because it is only through faith and engagement that we will end up with a fairer system," said Morales-Doyle.

The Census

The constitutionally required census is among the most important civil rights issues of our day.
—The Leadership Conference on Civil and Human Rights[20]

The tradition of counting every person in the United States is enshrined in Article 1, Section 2 of the U.S. Constitution: "Enumeration shall be made within three Years after the first Meeting of the Congress of the United States, and within every subsequent Term of ten Years."[21]

The census aims to provide a snapshot of all people living in the United States on April 1 of every year that ends in zero. Lodged within the U.S. Department of Commerce, the Bureau of the Census directs the count and works with state, local, and community organizations to promote universal participation. The bureau describes the census as "the largest mobilization and operation conducted in the United States," requiring years of research and methods and infrastructure development to ensure a complete and accurate count.[22]

Despite the stated goal of counting every person, large groups of Americans were excluded from the census for many years. Officially, these people did not exist. Until 1870, African Americans were counted as only three-fifths of a person for purposes of Congressional representation,[23] a policy designed to increase the power of slaveholding states. Native people living in the general population were not counted at all until 1860, and those living on reservations have been counted only since 1900.[24]

Today, many people still go uncounted for a variety of other reasons. The Census Bureau designates groups as "hard to count" if they meet specified criteria for being hard to locate, hard to contact, hard to persuade, or hard to interview.[25] For example, some potential respondents do not fully understand the purpose of the census and do not see its relevance to their lives. Others do not receive census notices because they lack a permanent address or move frequently or they refuse to participate, sometimes based on concerns of how the information will be used.

Inaccurate census counts threaten democracy by skewing power. The count drives the number of seats each state receives in the U.S. House of Representatives, how those seats are distributed within the state, and the number of Electoral College representatives allocated to each state. Incorrect counts give some states more than their share of representation, and therefore greater influence in policy development, while other states receive less than their share. These inequities last for 10 years, until the next census.

Inaccurate counts also create disparities, as census data drive the allocation of federal resources for schools, health clinics, student aid, and other purposes.[26] "In fiscal year 2017, more than 300 federal spending programs relied on 2010 census-derived data to distribute $1.5 trillion to state and local governments, nonprofits, businesses, and households," according to an analysis by the George Washington University Counting for Dollars 2020 project.[27] Here, too, some states and communities get too much and others too little when the census counts are wrong.

Discouraging Census Participation

While garnering less public interest than presidential elections, census outcomes have a powerful impact on health, equity, and racial justice. Many of the barriers and misinformation campaigns aimed at deterring people from voting also dissuade them from completing the census and require similar civic engagement strategies to overcome.

> *Civic engagement helps us understand the "why" behind actions we take—*
> *why we vote, why we care about the census.*
>
> —Iyanrick John

As a former policy strategist for the Asian & Pacific Islander American Health Forum, Iyanrick John applied his health policy training to an organization with a civic engagement agenda that includes building coalitions and addressing barriers to census participation. Systemic barriers to obtaining an accurate count include inadequate sensitivity to the cultural history of some subgroups of Americans, limited investment in educating communities about the census, and lack of funding to engage those who have historically been excluded from civic life. "Race, class, and politics all come into play with the census," observed the NAACP's Jamal Watkins. "When we talk to our communities about the census, we are talking to an audience that feels completely disconnected from the benefits of our democracy, from our country."

Many potentially hard-to-reach census participants are also vulnerable to misinformation that instills fear. Proposals to include a citizenship question on the 2020 census, for example, generated anxiety among immigrants and others that census information would be used to track their whereabouts and punish them. While the U.S. Supreme Court prohibited inclusion of that question, and activists attempted to allay the fear, polls reported that more than 50% of people continued to believe it would be part of the census.[28]

Counting People During a Pandemic

As COVID-19 spread through the country, the 2020 census shifted to an emphasis on online responses, making participation harder for residents who lack broadband access—a disproportionately low-income and rural population—and for those who are unfamiliar with completing online questionnaires.

Concerns about conducting the 2020 census in the midst of COVID-19 also reverberated through the White House, the Census Bureau, Congress, civil rights organizations, and activists across the country. Intensive community-based canvassing efforts were replaced with hastily developed online alternatives as Census Bureau analysts began working primarily from home.

Frequent policy and deadline changes, proposed to accommodate concerns about the pandemic, instead created confusion and new barriers. In response, community members, nonprofit organizations, and public interest legal firms mounted educational, advocacy, and legal campaigns to ensure that people were not discouraged from participating in the census, but the process remained anything but smooth.

In April 2020, President Trump declared that the census count would be extended from the end of July until the end of October, a move that required Congressional approval and funds.[29] Given the urgency to recoup ground lost during the early days of the pandemic, the Census Bureau began operating under the president's declaration, assuming that approval would be forthcoming. The House of Representatives authorized the extension, but the Senate never acted on it.

In early August, testifying that they had been directed to shorten the proposed counting period in order to meet the end-of-year deadline for reporting results, Census Bureau officials announced that counting would end on September 30. A lower court blocked that decision after hearing concerns that an abbreviated schedule would result in significant undercounting and errors. Two weeks later, the U.S. Supreme Court overturned the lower court, ruling that the count could end on October 15. Ultimately that is what happened.[30]

At the end of April 2021, the Census Bureau released the first population count from the census, including the reapportionment of Congressional seats.[31] Starting with the 2022 midterm elections, Texas will gain two seats and five other states will gain one. Seven states will lose one seat. Data used to redraw Congressional districts within each state were made public in August 2021,[32] which created significant challenges to the requirement that new districts be developed before the midterm election.

Although the census doesn't generally foster rallies or marches, all of these events threatened its accuracy and comprehensiveness. When the integrity of the census is compromised, its role as a primary tool of informed democracy is severely diminished.

Racial Diversity and the Census

One of the fundamental roles of the census is to paint a demographic portrait of Americans in all of their diversity. Respondents declare themselves to be members of one or more of the racial groups listed in the survey. The more choices people are offered, the more likely the count will accurately reflect the ways in which they self-identify, explained John. "The racial categories included in the census questionnaire generally reflect a social definition of race in this country and not an attempt to define race biologically, anthropologically, or genetically," according to Census Bureau survey guidance.[33]

Asian Americans, Native Hawaiians, and Pacific Islanders: Undercounted and Invisible

Asian Americans, Native Hawaiians, and Pacific Islanders comprise a diverse group of people who come from more than 50 countries across our largest continent of Asia and from multiple islands. They have unique cultural and historical profiles but have historically received less policy attention than other populations. Researchers and policymakers often aggregate people from these countries and islands into a small number of very large groups, thereby masking important differences among them that lead to policies that fail to recognize the unique characteristics, strengths, and needs of each.

The Census Bureau provides the following definitions:[34]

- **Asians** are individuals with origins in any of the original peoples of the Far East, Southeast Asia, or the Indian subcontinent (the countries are specified in the definition).
- **Native Hawaiians and Other Pacific Islanders** descend from any of the original peoples of Hawaii, Guam, Samoa, or other Pacific Islands (those islands are specified in the definition).

In 2019, the United States was home to 18.6 million Asians[35] and 628,000 Native Hawaiians and Other Pacific Islanders, according to data from the American Community Survey[36], a separate survey conducted by the Census Bureau each year.[37] Asians identifying as Indian and Chinese each represent more than 4 million people and those identifying as Filipino represent nearly 3 million.

Survey respondents also indicate where they live, and their answers indicate that Asians and Native Hawaiian and Other Pacific Islanders increasingly live in geographically dispersed regions that John describes as "growing mid-major cities." Four states—Indiana, North Carolina, Texas, and Utah—saw their Asian American populations increase by more than 40% between 2010 and 2017.[38] Five other states—New York, Pennsylvania, Rhode Island, South Dakota, and Wyoming—doubled their Native Hawaiian and Other Pacific Islander population during the same period.

Asian Americans are especially likely to be underrepresented or misrepresented in census counts. The 2020 Census Barriers, Attitudes, and Motivators Study of more than 17,000 White, Black, Hispanic, and Asian respondents revealed some troubling perceptions of the 2020 census and barriers to participation:[39]

- Only 55% of Asians said they were extremely or very likely to complete the census (compared with 69% of Whites, 65% of Hispanics[40] of any race, and 64% of Blacks).

- Nearly twice as many Asians (38%) as Blacks and Whites (20% and 19% respectively) said they were not at all or not too familiar with the census. Nearly one-third (30%) of Hispanics said they were not familiar with the census.
- Fully 42% of Asians were extremely or very concerned that their answers would not be kept confidential (compared with 38% of Blacks, 35% of Hispanics, and 24% of Whites).

Some challenges in fully and accurately counting Asian Americans and Native Hawaiians and Other Pacific Islanders stem from their personal circumstances. According to a 2018 Urban Institute report about Asian Americans, for example:[41]

- About one-third (32%) of Asians living in the United States are not U.S. citizens.
- Asians account for 14% of people without documentation.
- More than one-third (37%) of Asian Americans arrived in the United States after 2010 and have not had prior experience with the census.
- More than one-third (35%) have limited English proficiency and about 20% live in a household without an adult who speaks English well.
- Memories persist of the abuse of 1940 census data to target and incarcerate Japanese Americans in internment camps during World War II.

Limited internet access can also be a formidable barrier, John said, especially because census promotional material encouraged people to complete their 2020 questionnaires online. Other systemic challenges foster further barriers for Asian Americans (see Chapter 2). Long-standing racist attitudes have left scars that discourage census participation and that racism persists, most recently in the alarming increase of hate crimes against Asian Americans, and disgraceful references to COVID-19 as the "China virus" and "Kung Flu." By creating false perceptions and fomenting anger, they have helped to fuel a rising tide of discrimination,[42] a further barrier to civic engagement of any kind.

The extent to which census data are aggregated across people of different Asian origins has become salient in the public policy debate about balancing protecting privacy on one side and eliminating stereotypes on the other. The tendency to aggregate data perpetuates "a 'model minority' myth which suggests that Asian Americans have overcome their barriers and are thriving in American society," John said, noting that the myth is misleading and damaging. This stereotype leads policymakers to conclude that "Asian Americans merit neither resources nor attention as an ethnic minority group within the American population," according to a 2016 article appearing in *Ethnicity & Disease*.[43] The article continues, "Conversely, the model minority stereotype implies that minorities other than Asian Americans are stereotypically lazy, driving a wedge between Asian Americans and other ethnic minority groups."

Disaggregating data into smaller components poses its own challenges, however, yielding small samples that may generate privacy concerns or be too small to analyze accurately, John acknowledges. To address those challenges, data collected by subgroup can be retained for select internal analyses and then collapsed into larger categories for other analyses or public reporting. Another approach is to pool multiple small samples of data over time to discern patterns and trends. At least two RWJF projects aim to improve the collection and analysis of disaggregated data, including census data:

- The University of California, Los Angeles is sponsoring a Workshop Series, "Addressing Health Equity Through Data Disaggregation," to help people who use health data increase representation of population groups.
- The Asian & Pacific Islander Health Forum guided the work of a multiracial collaborative of racial justice groups to improve the collection, analysis, and reporting of disaggregated state-level race and ethnicity data.

Aggregation of census data has become embroiled in legal disputes and might be headed for the U.S. Supreme Court.[44] In an attempt to balance privacy concerns with sharing the demographic information required to establish federal policies, funding, and research, the Census Bureau has been drawing from a mathematical concept called "differential privacy." This introduces "noise" into the data, which makes them harder to exploit, but also makes the data unusable for small populations. Alabama filed a lawsuit to block the bureau from using differential privacy, and 16 other states have filed amicus briefs. Civil rights groups have also expressed concern and may file separate lawsuits.

Partnerships to Promote Census Participation

To overcome the many barriers to securing an accurate count of the population living in America, community and philanthropic organizations have developed a number of initiatives designed to drive broader census participation—and then to build on successes to pursue other community goals.

Two projects of the W.K. Kellogg Foundation's Racial Equity Anchor Collaborative, a coalition of national racial justice and civil rights organizations, highlight the power of partnerships as they engage people from diverse racial groups in civic activities. Both the NAACP and the Asian & Pacific Islander American Health Forum are members of the collaborative.

Mapping the Count

Mapping the Count is an NAACP-directed initiative that combines census data with community engagement to increase census participation in low-income and minority communities across the country.[45] The Mapping the Count data hub curated daily updates on the census response, matching data indicating areas with low response rates to in-house data about the racial and ethnic composition of those areas. NAACP staff then targeted those communities for extra attention, reaching out to local partners in those areas to do the legwork. "We turned census data into a tool that helped us engage people who would likely have been overlooked," explained Watkins.

My Family Matters, My Family Counts

My Family Matters, My Family Counts, a project of the Kellogg collaborative, developed community interventions to increase census participation in Florida and Michigan. The national partners created educational messages targeted to diverse communities, prepared toolkits for local agencies, and provided national and local trainings, initially through in-person convenings and then as virtual events during the pandemic. The dual goals were to promote census participation and to highlight shared interests among people of different backgrounds. "Communities are more alike than they are different. We should emphasize and foster these commonalities, and not allow communities to be falsely divided," John said.

In Miami, agencies representing Asian Americans and Pacific Islanders worked together with those serving Haitian and Nigerian communities to maximize their participation in the census and to build enduring cross-racial relationships to tackle future projects. Among other activities, they put census information into packages of food and other resources being distributed at local food drives, meeting immediate community needs as they encouraged residents to respond to the census.

A Final Word

History has taught us that the path to democracy has often been forged by those who have been excluded from it. People denied rights as basic as the right to vote or the right to be counted have used the tools of civic engagement to advocate for an equitable society characterized by strong communities, commitment to change, and a seat at the table for everyone.

The need for that work has never stopped. Over the centuries, American institutions and its people have been sorely tested, standing up again and again to defend democracy and push it closer to a vision that remains unrealized, especially for its Black and Brown communities. The global pandemic, the stark visibility of systemic racism, increasing income inequality, and the violent aftermath of a contentious election are testing us once again.

The contributors to this chapter have highlighted two fundamental tools of civic engagement that are foundational to democracy and paint a stark picture of how they are threatened. At the same time, they offer inspiration and motivation to continue the work, which is always urgent yet never finished, as Pulitzer Prize–winning poet and writer Archibald MacLeish so eloquently said: "Democracy is never a thing done. Democracy is always something that a nation must be doing."

Epilogue

RWJF Looks Toward the Future

Following the 2020 RWJF *Sharing Knowledge* conference, the unprecedented challenges described in this book—the disparate consequences of the COVID-19 pandemic, the murder of George Floyd and the police violence it displayed, and the economic crisis that was extreme in communities of color—became known in some circles as "the triple pandemic."[1]

Within RWJF we began to address this critical moment in a variety of ways. While recognizing that the concurrent crises garnered immediate headlines, the Foundation knew from decades of involvement with its grantees that neither racial injustice nor economic inequality was a sudden event. Rather, they were endemic, nurtured by systemic disparities that could not be addressed without tackling racism, poverty, powerlessness, and lack of access to good jobs, education, housing, and healthcare. Said RWJF's CEO Richard Besser, "The inequalities laid bare by COVID-19 simply flow from the existing pandemic of racism and racial violence we are witnessing today."[2]

In this critical moment, RWJF embraced what Besser described as "a window of opportunity" to address the challenges that racial justice and community activists have long highlighted. This crisis, he said, "is making an already unfair system even worse, and that is completely unacceptable. It is critical that we make real and lasting improvements through community action and public policy in the months and years to come. Otherwise, the world's richest nation will have failed its people."[3]

> *The urgency of the times requires us to act boldly, take risks, and to engage promptly.*
>
> —Richard Besser[4]

Necessary Conversations. Edited by: Alonzo L. Plough, Oxford University Press. © Robert Wood Johnson Foundation 2022.
DOI: 10.1093/ oso/9780197641477.003.0019

In the weeks immediately after the conference and in the year that followed, RWJF took a series of steps that reflected actions and advocacy for and with the people most impacted—along with a stronger, more public voice against health and racial disparities.

The Foundation's Rapid Response

RWJF's response to COVID-19 began with two overarching realizations: the importance of having pre-existing relationships with local and regional foundations, especially those that support racial equity; and an awareness that immediate direct relief was needed, given what was sure to be the uneven impact of the pandemic. As a result, RWJF developed a $50 million rapid response relief package that it dispersed in just 15 days in April 2020.[5] Similar to rapid response grants initiated by the Foundation following catastrophic fires, flooding, or hurricanes, these grants, ranging from $10,000 to $4 million apiece, were designed to be spent within a matter of weeks to provide humanitarian assistance and direct housing, food, and economic support. The funding was meant to meet urgent needs without expectations for longer-term impacts.

About $20 million, or 40% of the total, went directly to 14 local and regional foundations already known to RWJF for their ability to quickly reach those most impacted and for their understanding of structural racism. This approach reflected recognition that as a national funder, RWJF was not equipped to do fast-turnaround grantmaking at the local level; it relied instead on foundation partners who knew the local context and local organizations and could mobilize to address urgent needs alongside a longer-term vision of racial equity and health equity.

Community Power Building

RWJF also understood that the rapid relief grants would not be sufficient to counter the influence of structural racism and racial inequities on health. A recurring theme in a growing body of work among RWJF grantees is the imperative of systems change and the role of the most impacted communities.

RWJF's Abbey Cofsky, managing director, program, felt that "a longer-term, strategic" question was in play at the Foundation as it considered how best to respond to the intertwined crises.

How do you then invest in the types of leaders, the types of organizations that will lift up the voices of those who have been historically marginalized?

> *How do you lift those voices up to identify what the solutions for their community should be?*
>
> —Abbey Cofsky

The answers can be found in a body of work that has been developing within RWJF for more than two decades: community power building, defined by RWJF as "the ability of communities most impacted by inequity to act together to voice their needs and hopes for the future and to collectively drive structural change, hold decision-makers accountable, and advance health equity."[6] The Foundation has in the past funded communities in power-building efforts to mitigate tobacco use and childhood obesity and, more recently, to improve community conditions and support workers' rights. (For more details see the Spotlight at the end of this chapter.)

When the pandemic hit, RWJF drew on lessons learned as it elevated its commitment to community power building. As Besser wrote in a July 2020 letter to the RWJF Board of Trustees: "It is time to take what we have learned from our work on building community power and deploy it with scale . . . to increase the ability of communities to wield power for health equity."

In the summer of 2020, the commitment to this work was cemented when the Foundation launched *Increasing Community Power*, a $90 million strategic program to enable an estimated 200 community organizations across the United States to take on issues that disproportionately impact people of color. The largest one-time strategic funding response in the Foundation's history, it reflects an evolving understanding of the role that community power building plays in advancing racial and health equity.

Slated to run for two years, RWJF organized its *Increasing Community Power* funding around three themes:[7]

- *Birth Equity and Justice for Women of Color*, which recognizes that the implicit bias and structural racism influencing maternal and infant health outcomes must be addressed (see Chapter 4). Acknowledging that RWJF is relatively new to the birth justice field, this effort supports established organizations, including SisterSong, Groundswell Fund, the Ms. Foundation for Women, and the National Birth Equity Collaborative, which will, among other initiatives, regrant funds to constituency-led, grassroots community groups.

  "America has a maternal health crisis, and it is rooted in our nation's long history of racism that persists to this day," co-wrote Stacey D. Stewart, president and CEO of the March of Dimes, and Richard Besser in a July 2021 opinion piece. "To achieve birth equity and justice—the idea that all who give birth should have healthy pregnancies, healthy babies, and the ability to thrive—we must dismantle the structural racism and health inequities that fuel these disparities."[8]

- *Housing Justice*, which recognizes that systemic racism in housing policies and practices fosters residential segregation and health disparities (see Chapter 9). This work will ensure that renters' priorities and needs are being honored in local decisions related to housing affordability, evictions, community conditions, and well-being while recognizing and building power among low-income renters who have experienced housing instability. Funding provided to national housing networks like Right to the City Alliance, People's Action Institute, the Center for Popular Democracy, and the Partnership for Working Families will support this work through local organizations.

- *Local Base-Building*, which seeks to build broad-based community power, with people of color, especially women, taking the lead. This effort is helping to grow the capacities of local organizations that organize and advocate for low-income community members (with a focus on youth and the South). Working with regional and national partners, these organizations are advancing policy, narrative, and systems changes across multiple issues, including housing, education, healthcare, and economic justice. Notably, the majority of each grant to national and regional networks like the Color of Change Education Fund, the National Domestic Workers Alliance, and the Georgia Strategic Alliance for New Direction and Unified Policies (Georgia STAND-UP) will be regranted to local affiliates, chapters, and partners to carry out the local base-building efforts.

- According to RWJF, "base-building is central to providing historically excluded populations with power, agency, and voice and requires an eco-system of capacities tailored to advance racial and health equity."[9]

By early 2021, RWJF had identified the national and regional organizations that would receive funding across these three programmatic areas and in turn support local entities and community efforts. This initiative, Besser explained, "will build the power of communities to press for change that will enhance racial equity, and ultimately build the kind of robust Culture of Health that we envision as a Foundation."

Building Better Data for Better Health

In concert with its efforts to build community power, RWJF recognized the immediate need for better public health and health-related data systems—another area of racial and health inequity brought into stark relief by the COVID-19 pandemic. Through *Transforming Public Health Data Systems to Advance Health Equity*, the Foundation allocated $10 million for nine months (September 2020 to April 2021) to fund "timely activities to support the transformation of public health and health-related data systems to improve health equity."

Specifically, this funding addresses the lack of racially disaggregated data, delays in data reporting, and limited data tracking and sharing across sectors by race, gender, and ethnicity—all factors that have contributed to the disproportionate impacts of COVID-19 on low-income communities and communities of color. To redress that, RWJF established a first-of-its-kind commission to reimagine how health data are collected, shared, and used, and to identify the public and private sector investments needed to modernize health data infrastructure and improve health equity. Led by Gail C. Christopher (a contributor to Chapter 1), this National Commission to Transform Public Health Data is charged with identifying how data can better illuminate the ways in which structural racism drives health inequities.

"We learned quickly that our ability to respond appropriately to the disparate impact of COVID-19 would be impeded by challenges with inconsistent data collection," wrote Christopher and Plough in a *Health Affairs* blog, describing the work on the new RWJF-funded commission. "Today the extent of the failure is widely known and alarming. While the current public health data system in the United States has historically faced challenges, the pandemic has shown that the data infrastructure is particularly deficient when it comes to protecting the most vulnerable."[10]

In its report[11], released in October 2021, the commission noted that "the current approach to data tells a story of disparities decontextualized from history and experience at aggregated levels that miss important dimensions of race, intersectionality, and place." To correct what it called "the urgency" of this deeply flawed data landscape, the commission recommended changes under three major themes:

- "Health equity and well-being narrative" to emphasize the importance of centering public health as the nation's pathway to better health and to promote the role of data in this process
- "Equitable governance, systems, and community engagement" partnerships to create a data system that understands what drives health
- "Measuring and addressing the health impact of systemic and structural racism."[12]

There is not only an urgent need for disaggregated data to better show inequities in outcomes, but also for data that can help explain why those inequities exist. COVID-19 has only put a glaring spotlight on gaps that have existed for far too long.

—Health Affairs blog, co-authored by Gail C.
Christopher and Alonzo Plough

Changing Conversations and Narratives

An unmistakable shift in tone in response to the structural racism and other intersectionalities was already evident at the Jackson conference. "In that setting, against the backdrop of building racial inequities and unease across the country, the conference had an urgency to it, a little anger or maybe a lot of anger," explained Plough. "As one of our presenters said, 'We lost our PG rating.'"
Yet the visibility and scale of the inequities laid bare by the pandemic was startling even for those already focused on health equity. Shaping a response required new conversations and new narratives, within RWJF and across the country.

"There's an awakening about racial equity and health equity because of the disproportionate impact that has been made evident through the pandemic," said Julie Morita, MD, RWJF's executive vice president. "And it's not just that it's communities of color who are being disproportionately impacted—it's the *reasons* these communities of color are being disproportionately impacted. And that's the conversation that I don't think has happened widely in the past."

Much like its community power-building work, RWJF's commitment to stronger, more deliberate conversations about racism emerges from a long arc of grantee efforts to promote the narrative changes that now seem so urgent. For instance, Pop Culture Collaborative (PCC), a project supported by RWJF and other philanthropies, works with artists, scientists, social justice organizers, and strategists to shape stories that advance racial, gender, and economic justice. Part of that effort involves investing in new talent and entertainment outlets capable of delivering—and willing to deliver—those stories.[13] And at the University of Southern California Annenberg School for Communications and Journalism, RWJF funded the Center for Health Journalism's 2020 National Fellowship, providing 22 diverse journalists a chance to consider the social, racial, and economic inequities exposed by COVID-19.[14] This continues a series of RWJF grants to USC since 2011 aimed at embedding health and racial equity messages in media and entertainment.[15]

Leaders at RWJF, too, are increasingly engaged in narrative-changing conversations about racial equity, both in public and behind closed doors. When

Pulitzer Prize–winning journalist and author Nikole Hannah-Jones, a contributor to this book (see Chapter 1), was initially denied tenure at the University of North Carolina-Chapel Hill, Besser did not hesitate in June 2021 to write to the school's Board of Trustees to express the Foundation's concern and support for Hannah-Jones, and to ask for reassurances that she was "being treated fairly and equitably."

(Citing racism and failed leadership, Hannah-Jones ultimately turned down a too-late offer of tenure at UNC and instead accepted a tenured position at Howard University, where she will launch a Center for Journalism and Democracy.[16])

As RWJF contemplates its evolving role in ongoing dialogue and research on structural racism's impact on health, it is also considering new approaches to measuring a Culture of Health. Instead of looking at disease indicators—"a kind of rear-view mirror measure," Plough said—RWJF is shifting to indicators that reflect what makes a community thrive. "As we broaden our thinking about equity and about what we aspire to be, we want to measure things that look at where we should be. Are communities thriving? How is our well-being? With a heightened awareness post-pandemic, our national measures may be changing."

Using Our Voice as Never Before

The shifts in RWJF's tone during the events of 2020 reflect both continuity and a deeper focus on its mission to address health disparities, advance solutions to fight racial and economic inequities, and pursue community empowerment.

"The Foundation was on a path toward addressing racial inequities and particularly structural racism before the pandemic hit," said Donald F. Schwarz, MD, senior vice president, program, at RWJF. Schwarz noted that a "considerable amount of work in our pipeline" already focused on racial equity and racial economic justice, targeting income and wealth gaps as well as inequitable housing, gentrification, and displacement in American cities." The Healthy Neighborhoods Equity Fund in Boston and the Living Cities collaboration of financial institutions and foundations, both funded by RWJF alongside other foundations, are two examples.

The changes that did occur reflected what Plough called "a change in inflection, because we were on this trajectory but we amped it up. We intensified it. We became more precise. We are now looking at racial equity with even a bigger and broader lens in all of our work. We've always known that you can't really talk about health inequity without talking about racial inequity, but now we are being more exact about the connection between the two and we are using our voice in a different way."

The Foundation's commitment to speaking out about inequities is likely to grow stronger with time. "We've talked about the importance of equity—and we mean everyone having a fair and just opportunity for health and well-being," said Besser. "What has become clearer and more explicit in our work is the essential need to talk about racial equity, and the role that structural racism plays in our society as a barrier to health for so many. I think that the transition, the increased focus on racial equity, has accelerated due to the experiences of 2020 and through the COVID-19 pandemic, the economic crisis, and the movement for racial justice."

> *The Foundation has become much more explicit about the role of racial equity and racial justice in providing opportunity for health or creating barriers to achieve that.*
> —Richard Besser

Spotlight

Building on Past Work to Seize a Moment

RWJF's immediate and long-term responses to the challenges laid bare by the events of 2020 built on a body of work that has existed for nearly two decades at the Foundation: community power building. These efforts to improve health led to programs designed to address tobacco cessation, lack of access to healthcare, childhood obesity, and, more recently, school discipline and worker rights. A few examples:[1]

- In 2004, RWJF funded Tobacco Policy Change, which worked intensively with low-income and Native American communities and with communities of color to build coalition campaigns for tobacco control policies. The Foundation sought out agencies that had credibility within their communities even if they lacked expertise in health, including groups that had worked on safety, Main Street redevelopment, and housing.
- In 2008, RWJF supported the Praxis Project and created Communities Creating Healthy Environments to "apply the principles and practices of community organizing and social justice to reversing childhood obesity in communities of color."[2]
- In 2011, RWJF worked with the Funders' Collaborative on Youth Organizing to increase the resources available to young people of color for social justice organizing and to promote the leadership of low-income young people.
- Since 2011, RWJF's Voices for Healthy Kids initiative has made it easier for all children to eat healthy foods and be active, and Forward Promise has strengthened communities that raise and empower boys and young men of color.
- In 2014, RWJF announced its vision to build a Culture of Health "that provides everyone in America a fair and just opportunity for health and

Necessary Conversations. Edited by: Alonzo L. Plough, Oxford University Press. © Robert Wood Johnson Foundation 2022. DOI: 10.1093/ oso/9780197641477.003.0020

well-being." Three years later, the Foundation added health equity to this vision. Health equity "requires removing obstacles to health such as poverty, discrimination, and their consequences, including powerlessness and lack of access to good jobs with fair pay, quality education and housing, safe environments, and healthcare."[3] Reflecting decades of experience tackling some of the most profound economic, social, and cultural challenges facing the country, the Culture of Health vision illustrates RWJF's commitment to equity, and to addressing racism as a prerequisite to equity.

- Launched in January 2016 in partnership with other philanthropic foundations, SPARCC (Strong, Prosperous and Resilient Communities Challenge) is a multiyear community development initiative supported by RWJF in six regions of the country to ensure that "public investments in the built environment reduce racial disparities, build a Culture of Health, and respond to the climate crisis." Among its many strategies, SPARCC stresses the need to "shift power and decision-making practices" to those most impacted.

- In 2019, RWJF continued its focus on capacity building with national civic and faith organizations, including NAACP, UnidosUS (formerly National Council of La Raza), Faith in Action (formerly PICO National Network), and the YMCA.

- In 2019, RWJF launched Lead Local: Exploring Community-Driven Change and the Power of Collective. The program is designed to explore this question: How does community power catalyze, create, and sustain conditions for healthy communities? As an example, one grant allowed three large community organizations to come together to advance a city-funded housing trust fund that provided affordable homes for low-income families at risk of displacement.

NOTES

Introduction

1. Besser R. Opinion: As coronavirus spreads, the bill for our public health failures is due. *Washington Post.* March 5, 2020. https://www.washingtonpost.com/opinions/as-coronavirus-spreads-the-bill-for-our-public-health-failures-is-due/2020/03/05/9da09ed6-5f10-11ea-b29b-9db42f7803a7_story.html
2. To understand more about this universalist perspective, read: McGee H. *The Sum of Us: What Racism Costs Everyone and How We Can Prosper Together.* 2021. Penguin Random House, New York, NY

Prologue

1. Boler J. Slave resistance in Natchez, Mississippi (1719–1861). Mississippi History Now. 2006.
2. U.S. Census. QuickFacts Mississippi. *https://www.census.gov/quickfacts/MS*
3. Ablaza K. 10 things you should know about Natchez on its 300th birthday. Mississippi Today. August 2, 2016. *https://mississippitoday.org/2016/08/02/10-things-you-should-know-about-natchez-on-its-300th-birthday/*
4. Phillips J. Reconstruction in Mississippi (1865–1876). Mississippi History Now. *http://www.mshistorynow.mdah.ms.gov/articles/204/reconstruction-in-mississippi-1865-1876*
5. Black Codes. History.com. *https://www.history.com/topics/black-history/black-codes*
6. *The Mississippi Delta—Where "Cotton Was King."* American Experience (PBS). *https://www.pbs.org/wgbh/americanexperience/features/emmett-sharecropping-mississippi/*
7. Irwin JR, O'Brien AP. Economic progress in the postbellum South? African American incomes in the Mississippi Delta, 1880–1910. *Explorations in Economic History.* 2001;38(1):166–180.
8. https://www.alcorn.edu/uploaded/files/oaa/Mississippi_Constitution.pdf
9. Black population by state. World Population Review. *https://worldpopulationreview.com/state-rankings/black-population-by-state*
10. USDA Economic Research Service. Percent of total population in poverty. *https://data.ers.usda.gov/reports.aspx?ID=17826#P47e289f3f7214c2da3e3a1d3b197562a_3_506iT5*
11. Rural Health Information Hub. Mississippi. *https://www.ruralhealthinfo.org/states/mississippi#:~:text=According%20to%20the%20USDA%20Economic,urban%20areas%20of%20the%20state*
12. Mississippi Department of Agriculture and Commerce. Agency information. *https://www.mdac.ms.gov/agency-info/mississippi-agriculture-snapshot/*
13. Feeding America. Hunger in Mississippi. *https://www.feedingamerica.org/hunger-in-america/mississippi#:~:text=In%20Mississippi%2C%20559%2C350%20people%20are,meal%20in%20Mississippi%20is%20%242.90*

14. Center on Budget and Policy Priorities. Mississippi Supplemental Nutrition Assistance Program. January 15, 2021. *https://www.cbpp.org/sites/default/files/atoms/files/snap_factsheet_mississippi.pdf*

15. United Way of the National Capital Area. Mapping the effect of COVID-19 on food insecurity across the country. October 19, 2020. *https://unitedwaynca.org/stories/food-insecurity-statistics/*

16. Harris B. How Mississippi's districts are separated into haves and have-nots. Hechinger Report. January 24, 2020. *https://hechingerreport.org/economic-segregation-how-mississippis-districts-are-separated-into-haves-and-have-nots/*

17. Congressional Research Service. The 10-20-30 provision: Defining persistent poverty counties. February 24, 2021. *https://fas.org/sgp/crs/misc/R45100.pdf*

18. County Health Rankings and Roadmaps. *https://www.countyhealthrankings.org/*

19. Persistent Poverty Working Group. *https://fahe.org/wp-content/uploads/PPWG-Document.pdf*

20. U.S. Department of the Treasury. What are CDFIs? *https://www.cdfifund.gov/sites/cdfi/files/documents/cdfi_infographic_v08a.pdf*

21. Hope Credit Union. *https://hopecu.org*

22. National Credit Union Administration. What is a credit union? *https://www.mycreditunion.gov/about-credit-unions/credit-union-different-than-a-bank*

23. Hope Credit Union. *www.hopecu.org/about*

24. Hope Credit Union. *https://hopecu.org/stories/hope-makes-home-sweet-again/*

25. Hope Credit Union. Transformational deposits. *https://hopecu.org/manage/media/Transformational-Deposits-TD-06-v1.pdf*

26. Mississippi Poor People's Campaign. *https://www.poorpeoplescampaign.org/committee/mississippi/*

27. http://onevoicems.org

28. Cascio E. What happened when kindergarten went universal? *Education Next*. 2010;10(2). *https://www.educationnext.org/what-happened-when-kindergarten-went-universal/*

29. Williams TMH. An exploration of how second-grade students' reading attitudes and motivations for reading are affected through family involvement via the Reading Book Satchels program. Doctoral dissertation, University of Southern Mississippi, 2003.

30. Mississippi Department of Education. Mississippi Family Engagement Framework and Toolkit. *https://www.mdek12.org/sites/default/files/final_ms_family_engagement_framework_final_1.pdf*

31. Carey G. Language gap between rich and poor children begins in infancy, Stanford psychologists find. *Stanford Report*. September 25, 2013. *https://news.stanford.edu/news/2013/september/toddler-language-gap-091213.html*

32. Mississippi Department of Education. MKAS² Kindergarten Readiness Assessment Update. May 21, 2015. *https://www.mdek12.org/sites/default/files/kra-sbe-preso-2015-05-21.pdf*

33. Mississippi Department of Education. Kindergarten Readiness Assessment Results. October 29, 2019. *https://www.mdek12.org/sites/default/files/Offices/MDE/OEA/OPR/2020/fall-2019-kindergarten-readiness-results_final_10.29.19.pdf*

34. Mississippi Department of Education. 2017-2018 Kindergarten Readiness Assessment Results. July 2018. *https://www.mdek12.org/sites/default/files/Offices/MDE/OEA/OPR/2018/2018_KRA_Results_KG_FY2018_Post-test_Final.pdf*

35. Skinner K. Who's teaching Mississippi's children? A deep dive into race, gender of state's educators. Mississippi Today. September 6, 2019. *https://mississippitoday.org/2019/09/06/whos-teaching-mississippis-children-a-deep-dive-into-teacher-demographics/*

Chapter 1

1. Linnean Society of London. Linnaeus and race. *https://www.linnean.org/learning/who-was-linnaeus/linnaeus-and-race*

2. U.S. National Library of Medicine. The world of Shakespeare's humors. *https://www.nlm.nih.gov/exhibition/shakespeare/fourhumors.html*

3. National Human Genome Research Institute. What is the Human Genome Project? *https://www.genome.gov/human-genome-project/What*

4. Human genomes, public and private. *Nature.* 2001;409:745. *https://doi.org/10.1038/35057454*

5. National Human Genome Research Institute. Race. *https://www.genome.gov/genetics-gloss ary/Race* Accessed December 26, 2020.

6. Urging the establishment of a United States Commission on Truth, Racial Healing, and Transformation. Congress.gov. *https://www.congress.gov/bill/116th-congress/house-concurr ent-resolution/100* Accessed August 19, 2021.

7. Hannah-Jones N. The 1619 Project. *New York Times Magazine.* August 18, 2019, p. 16.*https://www.nytimes.com/interactive/2019/08/14/magazine/black-history-american-democracy.html*

8. Hannah-Jones, 2019, p. 10.

9. The 1619 Project. *New York Times Magazine. https://www.nytimes.com/interactive/2019/08/14/magazine/1619-america-slavery.html* Accessed February 1, 2021.

10. Blackwell E. Texas pushes to obscure the state's history of slavery and racism. *New York Times.* May 20, 2021. *https://www.nytimes.com/2021/05/20/us/texas-history-1836-project.html*

11. https://apnews.com/article/florida-race-and-ethnicity-government-and-politics-education-74d0af6c52c0009ec3fa3ee9955b0a8d

12. Hannah-Jones N. What is owed. *New York Times Magazine.* June 28, 2020, p. 34. *https://www.nytimes.com/interactive/2020/06/24/magazine/reparations-slavery.html*

13. Hannah-Jones, 2020, p. 52.

14. Hannah-Jones, 2020, p. 34.

15. Hannah-Jones, 2020, p. 52.

16. Hannah-Jones, 2020, p. 52.

17. Hannah-Jones, 2020, p. 52.

18. NAACP. About NAACP. *https://naacp.org/about-us/* Accessed December 29, 2020.

19. Kahlenberg RD. An economic fair housing act. The Century Foundation. August 3, 2017. *https://tcf.org/content/report/economic-fair-housing-act/?agreed=1&agreed=1* Accessed January 2, 2021.

20. Exploring Constitutional Conflicts. Separate but equal: The road to *Brown. http://law2. umkc.edu/faculty/projects/ftrials/conlaw/sepbutequal.htm* Accessed January 3, 2021.

21. *Milliken v. Bradley*, 418 U.S. 717 (1974). Justia. *https://supreme.justia.com/cases/federal/us/418/717/*

22. García E. Schools are still segregated, and Black children are paying a price. Economic Policy Institute. February 12, 2020. *https://files.epi.org/pdf/185814.pdf*

23. Shapiro E. Only 7 Black students got into Stuyvesant, N.Y.'s most selective high school, out of 895 spots. *New York Times.* March 18, 2019. *https://www.nytimes.com/2019/03/18/nyregion/black-students-nyc-high-schools.html*

24. Mervosh S. How much wealthier are White school districts than nonwhite ones? $23 billion, report says. *New York Times.* February 27, 2019. *https://www.nytimes.com/2019/02/27/education/school-districts-funding-white-minorities.html*

25. Johnson D. When it comes to Covid-19, another case of white flight. CNN. May 11, 2020. *https://www.cnn.com/2020/05/11/opinions/covid-19-case-white-flight-johnson/index.html*

26. Aubrey A. CDC hospital data point to racial disparity in COVID-19 cases. NPR. April 8, 2020. *https://www.npr.org/sections/coronavirus-live-updates/2020/04/08/830030932/cdc-hospital-data-point-to-racial-disparity-in-covid-19-cases* Accessed January 13, 2021.

27. Aubrey, 2020.

28. Johnson, 2020.

29. Johnson, 2020.

30. Hannah-Jones, 2020, p. 53.

31. Associated Press. Evanston, Illinois, becomes first U.S. city to pay reparations to Black residents. NBC News. March 23, 2021. *https://www.nbcnews.com/news/us-news/evanston-illinois-becomes-first-u-s-city-pay-reparations-blacks-n1261791*

Chapter 2

1. *Decolonize Justice.* Latino Justice. January 31, 2020. *https://www.youtube.com/watch?v=GLfSYjpJ0PI*

2. Perry AM. School dress and grooming codes are the new "Whites-only" signs. The Brookings Institute, February 20, 2020. *https://www.brookings.edu/blog/brown-center-chalkboard/2020/ 02/14/school-dress-and-grooming-codes-are-the-new-whites-only-signs/*

3. LatinoJustice. National poll shows Latinos are concerned about police violence, feel less safe under Trump but insist on increased spending on rehabilitation instead of more funding for prisons or police. January 2017. *https://www.latinojustice.org/en/news/ national-poll-shows-latinos-are-concerned-about-police-violence-feel-less-safe-under-trump*

4. Light MT, He J, Robey JP. Comparing crime rates between undocumented immigrants, legal immigrants and native-born US citizens in Texas. *Proc Natl Acad Sci USA.* 2020;117(51):32340–32347. *https://www.pnas.org/content/117/51/32340*

5. Gonazalez-Barrera A. Hispanics with darker skin are more likely to experience discrimination than those with lighter skin. Pew Research Center. July 2, 2019. *https://www.pewresearch.org/ fact-tank/2019/07/02/hispanics-with-darker-skin-are-more-likely-to-experience-discrimination- than-those-with-lighter-skin/*

6. Gernand B. Numbers tell a story. Chocktaw Nation. *https://www.choctawnation.com/ numbers-tell-story*

7. Reclaiming Native Truth. Research Findings: Compilation of All Research. June 2018. *https://www.firstnations.org/publications/compilation-of-all-research-from-the-reclaiming- native-truth-project/*

8. Shear SB, Knowles RT, Soden GJ, Castro AJ. Manifesting destiny: Re/presentations of Indigenous peoples in K–12 U.S. history standards. *Theory & Research in Social Education.* 2015;43(1):68–101. doi:10.1080/00933104.2014.999849.

9. Leavitt PA, Covarrubia R, Perez YA, Fryberg SA. Frozen in time: The impact of Native American media representations on identify and self-understanding. *J Soc Issues.* 2015;71(1):39–53. doi:10.1111/josi.12095.

10. Leavitt et al., 2015.

11. Reclaiming Native Truth. Research Findings: Compilation of All Research. June 2018. *https:// illuminatives.org/wp-content/uploads/2018/04/FullFindingsReport-screen-spreads.pdf?x18008*

12. Estus J. Study finds only harmful effects from Native-themed mascots. Indian Country Today. *https://indiancountrytoday.com/news/study-finds-only-harmful-effects-from-native-themed- mascots-Gr8ez-HtvkeB-Q5SPNhmhw*

13. Jin CH. 6 charts that dismantle the trope of Asian Americans as a model minority. May 25, 2021. NPR. *https://www.npr.org/2021/05/25/999874296/ 6-charts-that-dismantle-the-trope-of-asian-americans-as-a-model-minority*

14. Yi SS, Kown SC, Sacks R, Trinh-Shevrin C. Commentary: Persistence and health-related consequences of the model minority stereotype for Asian Americans. *Ethnicity & Disease.* 2016;26(1):133–138.*https://www.ncbi.nlm.nih.gov/pmc/articles/PMC4738850/*

15. Brockell G. The long, ugly history of anti-Asian racism and violence in the U.S. *Washington Post.* March 20, 2021. *https://www.washingtonpost.com/history/2021/03/18/ history-anti-asian-violence-racism/*

16. Shah M, Kauh T. How do we advance health equity for Asian Americans? RWJF blog. June 23, 2021. *https://www.rwjf.org/en/blog/2021/06/how-do-we-advance-health-equity- for-asian-americans.html*

17. Hswen Y, Xu X, Hing A, Hawkins JB, Brownstein JS, Gee GC. Association of #covid19 Versus #chinesevirus" with anti-Asian Sentiments on Twitter, March 9–23, 2020. *AM J Public Health.* May 2021. *https://ajph.aphapublications.org/doi/10.2105/AJPH.2021.306154*

18. Morita J. Commentary: Racism is the other virus sweeping America during this pandemic. *Chicago Tribune.* April 20, 2020.

19. Opinion: The surge of attacks against Asian Americans requires attention and swift solution. *Washington Post.* March 12, 2021.

20. In Atlanta, Biden condemns attacks on Asian-Americans. *New York Times.* March 20, 2021.

21. Shah M, Kauh T. How do we advance health equity for Asian Americans? RWJF blog. June 23, 2021. *https://www.rwjf.org/en/blog/2021/06/how-do-we-advance-health-equity- for-asian-americans.html*

22. Columbia Law School. Kimberlé Crenshaw on intersectionality, more than two decades later. *https://www.law.columbia.edu/news/archive/kimberle-crenshaw-intersectionality-more- two-decades-later*

23. Transgender Law Center. Trans Agenda for Liberation. *https://transgenderlawcenter.org/trans-agenda-for-liberation?emci=a938fcb2-b760-eb11-9889-00155d43c992&emdi=04306967-6061-eb11-9889-00155d43c992&ceid=8611836*

Chapter 3

1. Global Meaning Institute. Meaningology. *http://www.globalmeaninginstitute.com/meaning-u.html*
2. Pattakos A. The deeper meaning of authentic dialogue. *Psychology Today*. July 3, 2019. *https://www.psychologytoday.com/us/blog/the-meaningful-life/201907/the-deeper-meaning-authentic-dialogue*
3. National Museum of African American History and Culture. Talking about race. *https://nmaahc.si.edu/learn/talking-about-race*
4. McIntosh P. White privilege: Unpacking the invisible knapsack. *Peace and Freedom.* July/August 1989. *https://psychology.umbc.edu/files/2016/10/White-Privilege_McIntosh-1989.pdf*
5. DiAngelo R. White fragility. *Int J Critical Pedagogy.* 2011;3(3):54–57. *https://libjournal.uncg.edu/ijcp/article/viewFile/249/116*
6. Gleig A. Waking up to Whiteness and White privilege. *UCF Today*, University of Central Florida. October 7, 2020. *https://www.ucf.edu/news/waking-up-to-whiteness-and-white-privilege/*
7. Moniuszko S. How to talk to your family, friends about racism and white privilege. *USA Today.* July 6, 2020. https://www.usatoday.com/story/life/2020/07/06/how-to-guide-talk-racism-white-privilege-with-family-friends/3278514001/ Updated January 7, 2021.
8. The invisibility of White privilege with Brian Lowery, PhD. American Psychological Association, Episode 110, Speaking of Psychology podcast. July 2020. *https://www.apa.org/news/podcasts/speaking-of-psychology/white-privilege*
9. Loretta J. Ross. *www.Lorettajross.com*
10. South Carolina College of Arts and Sciences. The College of Arts and Sciences Collaborative on Race. *https://www.sc.edu/study/colleges_schools/artsandsciences/diversity/collaborative_on_race/index.php*
11. Courageous Conversation. *https://courageousconversation.com/about/*
12. Protestors' anger justified even if actions may not be. Monmouth University Polling Institute. June 2, 2020. *https://www.monmouth.edu/polling-institute/reports/monmouthpoll_us_060220/*

Spotlight

1. To form the Rx Racial Healing Circles™ Collaborative, Christopher worked in partnership with the Association of American Colleges & Universities, Community Action Partnership, American Public Health Association, National Collaborative for Health Equity, and her own Ntianu Garden: Center for Healing and Nature.
2. Garrett MT, Garrett JT, Brotherton D. Inner circle/outer circle: A group technique based on Native American healing circles. *Journal for Specialists in Group Work.* 2001;26(1):17–30. *https://doi.org/10.1080/01933920108413775*
3. McCraty R. Psychophysiological coherence: A proposed link among appreciation, cognitive performance, and health. Proceedings of the American Psychological Association 109th Annual Convention, Symposium on Gratitude and Positive Emotionality as Links Between Social and Clinical Science, San Francisco, CA, August 2001. *https://www.heartmath.org/research/research-library/abstracts/psychophysiological-coherence-a-proposed-link-among-appreciation/*
4. H.Con.Res.19-117th Congress (2021-22). Urging the establishment of a United States Commission on Truth, Racial Healing, and Transformation. *https://www.congress.gov/bill/117th-congress/house-concurrent-resolution/19/text*

Chapter 4

1. Infant mortality and African Americans. Office of Minority Health, U.S. Department of Health and Human Services, 2019. https://minorityhealth.hhs.gov/omh/browse.aspx?lvl=4&lvlid=23
2. Pregnancy Mortality Surveillance System. Centers for Disease Control and Prevention. https://www.cdc.gov/reproductivehealth/maternal-mortality/pregnancy-mortality-

surveillance-system.htm?CDC_AA_refVal=https%3A%2F%2Fwww.cdc.gov%2Freproduct ivehealth%2Fmaternalinfanthealth%2Fpregnancy-mortality-surveillance-system.htm

3. Report from nine Maternal Mortality Review Committees. Building U.S. capacity to review and prevent maternal deaths, 2018. Review to Action: Working Together to Prevent Maternal Mortality. *https://www.cdcfoundation.org/sites/default/files/files/ReportfromNineMMRCs.pdf*

4. Salam M. For Serena Williams, childbirth was a harrowing ordeal. She's not alone. *New York Times.* January 11, 2018. *https://www.nytimes.com/2018/01/11/sports/tennis/serena-williams-baby-vogue.html*

5. Purnell D. If even Beyoncé had a rough pregnancy, what hope do other Black women have? *The Guardian.* April 23, 2019. *https://www.theguardian.com/commentisfree/2019/apr/23/beyonce-pregnancy-black-women*

6. Melillo G. Racial disparities persist in maternal morbidity, mortality and infant health. *American Journal of Managed Care,* June 13, 2020. *https://www.ajmc.com/view/racial-disparities-persist-in-maternal-morbidity-mortality-and-infant-health*

7. Diabetes and African Americans. Office of Minority Health, U.S. Department of Health and Human Services, 2019. *https://minorityhealth.hhs.gov/omh/browse.aspx?lvl=4&lvlid=18*

8. Stroke and African Americans. Office of Minority Health, U.S. Department of Health and Human Services, 2020. *https://minorityhealth.hhs.gov/omh/browse.aspx?lvl=4&lvlid=28*

9. Heart disease and African Americans. Office of Minority Health, U.S. Department of Health and Human Services, 2020. *https://minorityhealth.hhs.gov/omh/browse.aspx?lvl=4&lvlid=19*

10. Cancer and African Americans. Office of Minority Health, U.S. Department of Health and Human Services, 2020. *https://minorityhealth.hhs.gov/omh/browse.aspx?lvl=4&lvlid=16*

11. Bailey AC. They sold human beings here. *New York Times.* February 12, 2020. *https://www.nytimes.com/interactive/2020/02/12/magazine/1619-project-slave-auction-sites.html*

12. Holland B. The "father of modern gynecology" performed shocking experiments on enslaved women. History.Com, 2018. *https://www.history.com/news/the-father-of-modern-gynecology-performed-shocking-experiments-on-slaves*

13. Ojanuga D. The medical ethics of the "father of gynaecology." *J Med Ethics.* 1993;19:28–31. *https://jme.bmj.com/content/medethics/19/1/28.full.pdf*

14. Lerner BH. Scholars argue over legacy of surgeon who was lionized, then vilified. *New York Times.* October 28, 2003. *https://www.nytimes.com/2003/10/28/health/scholars-argue-over-legacy-of-surgeon-who-was-lionized-then-vilified.html*

15. Michals D. Fannie Lou Hamer. National Women's History Museum, 2017. *https://www.womenshistory.org/education-resources/biographies/fannie-lou-hamer*

16. *Freedom Summer: Fannie Lou Hamer.* PBS American Experience: Women in American History. *https://www.pbs.org/wgbh/americanexperience/features/freedomsummer-hamer/*

17. *Laboring with Hope.* Six Dimensions, LLC, 2020. *https://www.laboringwithhope.com/*

18. Johnson JD, Asiodu IV, McKenzie CP, et al. Racial and ethnic inequities in postpartum pain evaluation and management. *Obstet Gynecol.* 2019;134(6):1155–1162. *https://pubmed.ncbi.nlm.nih.gov/31764724/*

19. Hoffman KM, Trawalter S, Axt JR, Oliver MN. Racial bias in pain assessment and treatment recommendations, and false beliefs about biological differences between Blacks and Whites. *Proc Natl Acad Sci USA.* 2016;113(16):4296–4301. *https://www.ncbi.nlm.nih.gov/pmc/articles/PMC4843483/*

20. Aronowitz SV, McDonald CC, Stevens RC, Richmond TS. Mixed studies review of factors influencing receipt of pain treatment by injured Black patients. *J Adv Nurs.* 2020;76(1):34–46. *https://onlinelibrary.wiley.com/doi/10.1111/jan.14215*

21. Geronimus AT. The weathering hypothesis and the health of African-American women and infants: Evidence and speculations. *Ethn Dis.* 1991;2(3):207–221. *https://pubmed.ncbi.nlm.nih.gov/1467758/*

22. DeVane-Johnson S, Giscombe CW, Williams II R, et al. A qualitative study of social, cultural, and historical influences on African American women's infant-feeding practices. *J Perinatal Educ.* 2018;27(2):71–85. *https://www.ncbi.nlm.nih.gov/pmc/articles/PMC6388681/*

23. Link BG, Phelan JC. Is racism a fundamental cause of inequalities in health? *Ann Rev Sociol.* 2015;41:311–330. *https://www.annualreviews.org/doi/pdf/10.1146/annurev-soc-073014-112305*

24. Crear-Perry J, Green C, Mahdi I. Birth equity requires hard truths and new leadership. Harvard Medical School: Center for Primary Care. January 14, 2021. *http://info.primarycare.hms.harvard.edu/blog/birth-equity-hard-truth-new-leadership*

25. Our history. SisterSong, Inc. *https://www.sistersong.net/mission*

26. What is reproductive justice? SisterSong, Inc. *https://www.sistersong.net/reproductive-justice*

27. Chadha N, Kane M, Lim B, Rowland B. Towards the abolition of biological race in medicine: Transforming clinical education, research and practice. Institute for Healing and Justice in Medicine, 2020. *https://www.instituteforhealingandjustice.org/executivesummary*

28. California Birth Equity Collaborative: Improving care, experiences and outcomes for Black mothers. California Maternal Quality Care Collaborative. *https://www.cmqcc.org/content/birth-equity*

29. Ruiz-Grossman S. California takes new steps to stop Black women from dying in childbirth. *Huffpost.* October 8, 2019. *https://www.huffpost.com/entry/california-bill-black-maternal-mortality_n_5d9cd594e4b06ddfc50f6f0e*

30. Supporting Mothers' Voices Driving Birth Equity in Tying the Voice of Patients to a Formal Quality Improvement Process. RWJF Grant Numbers: 76153 (12/15/2018–4/14/2020, $449,312) and 77392 (5/1/2020–10/31/2022, $965472).

31. Dehlendorf C, Akers AY, Borrero S, et al. Evolving the preconception health framework: A call for reproductive and sexual health equity. *Obstet Gynecol.* 2021;137(2):234–239. *https://journals.lww.com/greenjournal/Fulltext/2021/02000/Evolving_the_Preconception_Health_Framework__A.6.aspx*

32. Bohren MA, Hofmeyr GJ, Sakala C, et al. Continuous support for women during childbirth. *Cochrane Database Syst Rev.* 2017;7(7):CD003766. *https://pubmed.ncbi.nlm.nih.gov/28681500/*

33. *Lost Mothers: Maternal Mortality in The U.S.* NPR Special Series, 2017. *https://www.npr.org/series/543928389/lost-mothers*

34. Villarosa L. Why America's Black mothers and babies are in a life-or-death crisis. *New York Times Magazine.* April 11, 2018. *https://www.nytimes.com/2018/04/11/magazine/black-mothers-babies-death-maternal-mortality.html?searchResultPosition=1*

35. Maternal Mortality Review Committees. Guttmacher Institute. July 1, 2021. *https://www.guttmacher.org/state-policy/explore/maternal-mortality-review-committees#*

36. Mississippi Maternal Mortality Report: 2013–2016. Mississippi State Department of Health. April 2019. *https://msdh.ms.gov/msdhsite/_static/resources/8127.pdf*

37. Kieltyka L, Mehta P, Schoellmann K, Lake C. Louisiana Maternal Mortality Review Report 2011–2016. Louisiana Department of Health. August 2018. *https://ldh.la.gov/assets/oph/Center-PHCH/Center-PH/maternal/2011-2016_MMR_Report_FINAL.pdf*

38. Recommendation to the Governor to Reduce Maternal Mortality and Racial Disparities. New York State Taskforce on Maternal Mortality and Disparate Racial Outcomes. March 2019. *https://health.ny.gov/community/adults/women/task_force_maternal_mortality/docs/maternal_mortality_report.pdf*

39. Governor Cuomo signs legislation creating New York's Maternal Mortality Review Board. New York State. August 1, 2019. *https://www.governor.ny.gov/news/governor-cuomo-signs-legislation-creating-new-yorks-maternal-mortality-review-board*

40. Call for Office of Sexual and Productive Health and Wellbeing (OSRHW). National Birth Equity Collaborative. March 8, 2021. *https://birthequity.org/call-for-osrhw/*

41. Democratic senators ask Biden admin to create office focusing on reproductive health and wellbeing. The 19th, February 24, 2021. *https://19thnews.org/2021/02/democratic-senators-ask-biden-admin-to-create-office-focusing-on-reproductive-health-and-wellbeing/?utm_source=The+19th&utm_campaign=a1ce746196-19th-newsletters-daily&utm_medium=email&utm_term=0_a35c3279be-a1ce746196-381637492*

42. Reps. Kelly, Lee, DeGette lead letter asking Biden administration to establish Office of Sexual and Reproductive Health and Wellbeing. Office of Congresswoman Robin Kelly. March

18, 2021. *https://robinkelly.house.gov/media-center/press-releases/reps-kelly-lee-degette-lead-letter-asking-biden-administration-to*

43. Vogtman J. Undervalued: A Brief History of Women's Care Work and Child Care Policy in the United States. National Women's Law Center, 2017. *https://nwlc.org/wp-content/uploads/2017/12/final_nwlc_Undervalued2017.pdf*

44. Vogtman, 2017.

45. Child Care in Crisis: Stories from the Field. National Women's Law Center with a coalition of child-focused organizations, 2020. *https://nwlc.org/wp-content/uploads/2020/07/Child-Care-Storybook-Newest.pdf*

46. Jessen-Howard S, Workman S. Coronavirus pandemic could lead to permanent loss of nearly 4.5 million child care slots. American Progress. April 24, 2020. *https://www.americanprogress.org/issues/early-childhood/news/2020/04/24/483817/coronavirus-pandemic-lead-permanent-loss-nearly-4-5-million-child-care-slots/*

Spotlight

1. Howell EA. This intervention helps underserved women at Mount Sinai Hospital access needed postpartum care. Advancing Health Equity blog. June 5, 2017. *https://www.solvingdisparities.org/blog/intervention-helps-underserved-women-mount-sinai-hospital-access-needed-postpartum-care*

2. Howell EA, Balbierz A, Beane S, et al. Timely postpartum visits for low-income women: A health system and Medicaid payer partnership. *Am J Public Health.* 2020;110:S215–S218. *https://www.ncbi.nlm.nih.gov/pmc/articles/PMC7362690/*

Chapter 5

1. Hobor G, Plough A. Addressing mass incarceration to achieve health equity. *Am J Public Health.* 2020;110(S1):S13.

2. Gramlich J. Black imprisonment rate in the U.S. has fallen by a third since 2006. *FactTank: News in the Numbers,* Pew Research Center. May 6, 2020.

3. Acker J, Braveman P, Arkin E, Leviton L, Parsons J, Hobor G. *Mass Incarceration Threatens Health Equity in America.* Executive Summary. Princeton, NJ: Robert Wood Johnson Foundation, 2019.

4. Jones A, Sawyer W. Arrest, release, repeat: How police and jails are misused to respond to social problems. Press release, Prison Policy Initiative. August 2019.

5. Acker et al., 2019.

6. Gramlich, 2020.

7. Sawyer W, Wagner P. Mass incarceration: The whole pie 2020. Prison Policy Initiative. March 24, 2020.

8. Acker et al., 2019.

9. Hobor and Plough, 2020.

10. Gramlich, 2020.

11. Acker et al., 2019.

12. Casella J, Ridgeway J. America's worst prisons: Rikers Island. *Mother Jones.* May 14, 2013.

13. Hobor and Plough, 2020.

14. Statistics from interviews and conference presentations with Sherry Glied, PhD, and the revised 2020 report, *Quantifying Healthcare Needs and Use Among New Yorkers with Justice-Involvement,* by NYC Department of Health and Mental Hygiene, Mayor's Office of Criminal Justice, NYU Wagner Graduate School of Public Service.

15. New York City Department of Health and Mental Hygiene, Mayor's Office of Criminal Justice, and New York University Wagner Graduate School of Public Service. *Health Care Needs and Utilization Among New Yorkers With Criminal Justice System Involvement.* New York, New York, 2020.

16. Latest data shows Mississippi now ranked as second highest imprisoner in the nation. FWD. us. March 2, 2020.

17. Jay-Z and Yo Gotti file second lawsuit against Mississippi prisons. CNN.com. February 27, 2020.

18. Bor J, Venkataramani AS, Williams DR, Tsai AC. Police killings of unarmed black Americans have adverse effects on mental health among black American adults in the general population. *Lancet.* 2018;392(10144):P302–P310. *https://www.thelancet.com/journals/lancet/article/PIIS0140-6736(18)31130-9/fulltext*

19. Christopher G, Plough A. The role of racial justice in building a culture of health. *Health Affairs* blog. September 16, 2020.

20. Massoglia M, Pridemore WA. Incarceration and health. *Ann Rev Sociol.* 2015;41(1):291–310.

21. School-to-Prison Pipeline. ACLU, Juvenile Justice.

22. Buckwalter-Poza R, McElwee S. As pandemic rages, voters support releasing people from jails and prisons. *The Appeal.* February 5, 2021. Poll by Data for Progress and The Lab, a policy vertical of *The Appeal.*

23. Burkhalter E, Colón I, Derr B, et al. Incarcerated and infected: How the virus tore through the U.S. prison system. *New York Times.* April 11, 2021.

24. Melamed S. A man died after assault in Philly jail, where violence has surged under pandemic lockdown. *Philadelphia Inquirer.* January 20, 2021.

25. *The Belles,* Ear Hustle podcast, Radiotopia from PRX, a listener-supported network of independent, artist-owned podcasts.

26. Buckwalter-Poza and McElwee, 2021.

27. Herring T. Parole boards approved fewer releases in 2020 than in 2019. Prison Policy Institute. February 3, 2021.

28. Neil M. What the pandemic revealed about "progressive" prosecutors. *New York Times.* February 4, 2021.

29. Mississippi inmate deaths: Who died in 2021? *Clarion Ledger.* May 20, 2021.

30. Crown K. Reducing harsh sentencing goal of House bill to limit maximum sentencing requirement. *Jackson Free Press.* February 22, 2021.

31. Mower L, Taylor L. In Florida, the gutting of a landmark law leaves few felons likely to vote. ProPublica. October 7, 2020.

32. Hunter L. What you need to know about ending cash bail. Center for American Progress. March 16, 2020.

33. Egan L, Shabab R. Biden signs executive actions on racial equity. NBCNews.com. January 26, 2021.

34. Mississippi lawmakers advance commonsense criminal justice reform. Press release, FWD.us. February 11, 2021.

35. Mississippi governor signs bill to expand parole eligibility. WJTV. April 22, 2021.

36. Mass incarceration costs $182 billion every year, without adding much to public safety. Equal Justice Initiative. February 6, 2017.

37. Kushner R. Is prison necessary? Ruth Wilson Gilmore might change your mind. *New York Times Magazine.* April 17, 2019.

38. Acker et al., 2019.

Chapter 6

1. Budiman A. Key findings about U.S. immigrants. FactTank, Pew Research Center. August 20, 2020.

2. Wolf ZB. Yes, Obama deported more people than Trump but context is everything. CNN Politics. July 13, 2019; Guerrero J. 3 million people were deported under Obama. What will Biden do about it? *New York Times.* January 23, 2021; Stillman S. The race to dismantle Trump's immigration policies. *New Yorker.* February 1, 2021.

3. Budiman, 2020.

4. Passel J, Cohn D. Mexicans decline to less than half of the U.S. unauthorized immigrant population for the first time. Pew Research Center. June 12, 2019.

5. Castañeda H, Melo M. Health care access for Latino mixed-status families: Barriers, strategies and implications for reform. *Am Behav Sci.* 2014;58(14):1891–1909.

6. Logan R, Melo M, Castañeda H. Familial vulnerability: Impacts of legal status on mental health within mixed-status families. *Med Anthropol.* 2021;40(7):639–652.

7. Sammen J. The racism of US immigration policy. Center for Health Progress. August 1, 2018.

8. Not just a Latino issue: Undocumented Asians in America. Asia Society, Northern California, 2014.

9. Morita J. Commentary: Racism is the other virus sweeping America during this pandemic. *Chicago Tribune.* April 20, 2020.

10. U.S. Citizenship and Immigration Services. Public charge. *https://www.uscis.gov/green-card/green-card-processes-and-procedures/public-charge*

11. The 287(g) program: An overview. American Immigration Council, Fact Sheet. July 2, 2020.

12. Rhodes SD, Mann L, Simán FM, et al. The impact of local immigration enforcement policies on the health of immigrant Hispanics/Latinos in the United States. *Am J Public Health.* 2015;105(2):329–337. doi:10.2105/AJPH.2014.302218

13. Nichols V, LeBrón A, Pedraza F. Policing us sick: The health of Latinos in an era of heightened deportations and racialized policing. Political Science Now (American Political Science Association). May 16, 2018. *https://politicalsciencenow.com/policing-us-sick/*

14. LeBrón A, Schulz AJ, Gamboa C, et al. "They are clipping our wings": Health implications of restrictive immigrant policies for Mexican-origin women in a northern border community. *Race and Social Problems.* 2018;10(3):174–192.

15. Logan et al., 2021.

16. Castañeda and Melo, 2014.

17. Castañeda and Melo, 2014.

18. Logan et al., 2021.

19. Stillman, 2021.

20. Linton J, Griffin M, Shapiro A, Council on Community Pediatrics. Detention of immigrant children. *Pediatrics.* 2017;139(5):e20170483.

21. LeBrón AMW, Cowan K, Lopez WD, et al. The Washtenaw ID project: A government-issued ID coalition working toward social, economic, and racial justice and health equity. *Health Educ Behav.* 2019;46(1_suppl):53S–61S.

22. LeBrón A, Lopez WD, Cowan K, et al. Restrictive ID policies: Implications for health equity. *J Immigr Minor Health.* 2018;20(2):255–260.

23. LeBrón et al., 2019.

24. States offering driver's licenses to immigrants. National Conference of State Legislatures. February 8, 2021.

25. COVID-19 racial and ethnic health disparities. Centers for Disease Control and Prevention, updated December 10, 2020.

26. Centers for Disease Control and Prevention, 2020.

27. Johnson A. Death in the prime of life: Covid-19 proves especially lethal to younger Latinos. *Washington Post.* March 15, 2021.

28. Fricano M, Harlow J. A COVID crisis comes to light. *UCLA Magazine.* March 21, 2021.

29. Frederick W. What happens when people stop going to the doctor? We're about to find out. *New York Times.* February 22, 2021.

30. Johnson, 2021.

31. Hispanic adults in families with noncitizens disproportionately feel the economic fallout from COVID-19. The Urban Institute; summary at Coronavirus Pandemic (COVID-19), an RWJF Collection. May 1, 2020.

32. Lopez W, Kline N, LeBrón A, et al. Preventing the spread of COVID-19 in immigration detention centers requires the release of detainees. *Am J Public Health.* 2021;111(1):110–115.

33. Sacchetti M. ICE has no clear plan for vaccinating thousands of detained immigrants fighting deportation. *Washington Post.* March 12, 2021.

34. Colton H. Overwhelming public support for Albuquerque's $250K for migrants. KUNM Radio Weekend Edition. May 7, 2019.

35. Chelsea, Mass., creates COVID-19 hotel offering residents a safe, free place to isolate. RWJF Culture of Health Prize Winners feature. July 31, 2020.

36. Robert Wood Johnson Foundation awards communities the 2018 RWJF Culture of Health Prize. RWJF blog. September 18, 2018.

37. Shear M. Biden revokes Trump's pause on green cards. *New York Times.* February 24, 2021.

38. The Robert Wood Johnson Foundation, Grants #78332 and #78333. December 2020 and January 2021.

39. Federal policy recommendations to advance equity from the Robert Wood Johnson Foundation. *Health Policy in Brief,* the Robert Wood Johnson Foundation. January 19, 2021.
40. Grant No. 78305, Robert Wood Johnson Foundation: Creating a model for data-driven policymaking for Native Hawaiian and Pacific Islander populations in time of pandemic to help promote health equity.
41. Fricano and Harlow, 2021.
42. Shear M, Kanno-Youngs Z, Sullivan E. Young migrants crowd shelters, posing test for Biden. *New York Times.* April 10, 2021.
43. Castañeda and Melo, 2014.

Spotlight

1. Refugee Program, Illinois Department of Human Services, Refugee & Immigrant Services.
2. Illinois Welcoming Center (IWC), Illinois Department of Human Services, Refugee & Immigrant Services.

Chapter 7

1. *Bean v. Southwestern Waste Management Corporation,* widely recognized as the first lawsuit of its kind to use civil rights law to challenge environmental racism in the location of a waste facility. Filed in 1979, resolved in 1985.
2. Bullard R. Solid waste sites and the Houston Black community. *Sociological Inquiry.* 1983;53(2–3):273–288; Bullard RD. *Invisible Houston: The Black Experience in Boom and Bust.* College Station, TX: Texas A&M University Press, 1987.
3. Plough A. *Community Resilience: Equitable Practices for an Uncertain Future.* New York: Oxford University Press, 2021.
4. We may have just seen the world's highest recorded temperature ever. *The Guardian.* August 19, 2020.
5. Yoder K. The phrase "natural disaster" is going up in flames. Grist. September 16, 2020. *https://grist.org/climate/wildfires-the-phrase-natural-disaster-is-going-up-in-flames/*
6. Environmental justice and environmental racism, defined by Greenaction for Health and Environmental Justice. *https://greenaction.org/*
7. *Bean v. Southwestern Waste Management Corporation* (see note 1).
8. Bullard R. *Dumping in Dixie: Race, Class and Environmental Quality.* Taylor & Francis Group, 1990, 1994, 2000, and 2000; Routledge, 2018. Milton Park, Abingdon-on-Thames, Oxfordshire, England, UK
9. Chakaborty J, Collins T, Grinesk S. Exploring the environmental justice implications of Hurricane Harvey flooding in Greater Houston, Texas. *Am J Public Health.* 2018;109(2):244–250.
10. Bullard R, Wright B. *The Wrong Complexion for Protection: How the Government Response to Disaster Endangers African American Communities.* New York: New York University Press, 2012.
11. Plough, 2021.
12. Asthma and African Americans. U.S. Department of Health and Human Services, Office of Minority Health.
13. *Lancet* Countdown: Tracking Progress on Health and Climate Change. 2020.
14. Howell J, Elliott J. Damages done: The longitudinal impacts of natural hazards on wealth inequality in the United States. *Social Problems.* 2019;66(3):448–467.
15. 10 Things We Know about Race and Policing in the U.S. Pew Research Center. June 3, 2020.
16. Black Imprisonment Rate in the U.S. Has Fallen by a Third Since 2006. Pew Research Center. May 6, 2020.
17. Black people have been saying "we can't breathe" for decades. VICE. December 16, 2020. *https://www.vice.com/en/article/5dpy73/black-people-have-been-saying-we-cant-breathe-for-decades-robert-bullard*
18. Vicory J. Department of Health says Jackson is in violation of safe drinking water requirements. *Clarion Ledger.* July 18, 2018.

19. Water Equity slide revised, PolicyLink. March 2020.
20. *Closing the Water Access Gap in the United States: A National Action Plan*, a collaborative report by DigDeep Right to Water Project and U.S. Water Alliance, funded by the Robert Wood Johnson Foundation (Grant No. 76147), the United Methodist Committee on Relief, and the Water Foundation. 2019.
21. Chapman R. Advancing water equity for the nation's recovery and renewal. PolicyLink. May 27, 2020.
22. Flint Water Advisory Task Force Final Report. Commissioned by the Office of Governor Rick Snyder, State of Michigan. March 21, 2016.
23. Huang A. "Poster child" for environmental racism finds justice in Dickson, TN. Natural Resources Defense Council blog. December 8, 2011. *https://www.nrdc.org/experts/albert-huang/poster-child-environmental-racism-finds-justice-dickson-tn*
24. Water Equity and Climate Resilience Caucus, PolicyLink.
25. Water Equity and Climate Resilience Caucus, PolicyLink.
26. Chapman R. Coronavirus has laid bare the racial fault lines in access to clean, safe water. *The Guardian*. June 30, 2020.
27. Chapman, *The Guardian*, 2020.
28. Chapman, *The Guardian*, 2020.
29. Chapman, PolicyLink, 2020.
30. Colton H. NOAA investigates threats to fish stocks in a warmer Bering Sea. *Anchorage Daily News*. September 28, 2016.
31. Oscarville Tribal Climate Adaptation Plan, Oscarville Traditional Village, Alaska. Alaska Native Tribal Health Consortium and the Cold Climate Housing Research Center. 2018.
32. "Opportunities and challenges for washeterias in unpiped Alaska Native communities," Washeteria Technical Brief.
33. Gandhi P, Painter M. How communities are promoting health and responding to climate change. Culture of Health blog, Robert Wood Johnson Foundation, September 30, 2109. Grant No. 76579.
34. White-Newsome J, Meadows P, Kabel C. Bridging climate, health and equity: A growing imperative. *Am J Public Health*. 2018;108(Suppl 2):S72–S73.
35. Williams T. With a giant pledge, foundations spotlight a key niche for climate change philanthropy. Inside Philanthropy. September 12, 2018. *https://www.insidephilanthropy.com/home/2018/9/12/with-a-giant-pledge-foundations-spotlight-a-key-niche-for-climate-change-philanthropy*
36. The Intersection of Health, Equity and Climate Change, RWJF Health and Climate Solutions Initiative.
37. Climate Change, Health and Equity initiative, The Kresge Foundation.
38. HBCU Climate Change Consortium and HBCU-CBO Gulf Equity Consortium, Deep South Center for Environmental Justice. Funded by RWJF.
39. Eilperin J, Dennis B, Fears D. Biden to place environmental justice at the center of sweeping climate plan. *Washington Post*. January 27, 2021.
40. Eilperin et al., 2021.
41. Lavelle M. Environmental justice plays a key role in Biden's Covid-19 stimulus package. Inside Climate News. March 14, 2021. *https://insideclimatenews.org/news/14032021/environmental-justice-plays-a-key-role-in-bidens-covid-19-stimulus-package/*
42. Lavelle, 2021.

Chapter 8

1. While the cases discussed in this chapter focus on Black experiences, the dynamics and stakes apply to everyone in a racialized social system. We all stand to benefit from the promotion of justice and health equity, including the dominant group. For more information, read *Dying of Whiteness: How the Politics of Racial Resentment Is Killing America's Heartland*, a 2019 book by Jonathan M. Metzl.
2. For the first study of Jim Crow juvenile justice see Ward G. *The Black Child Savers: Racial Democracy and Juvenile Justice*. Chicago: University of Chicago Press, 2012. https://press.uchicago.edu/ucp/books/book/chicago/B/bo3752802.html

3. Ward noted, as an example, Metzl's work on how racial animus impacts health outcomes in White communities in Matzl, 2019.

4. Horrible tragedy. *Missouri Republican.* May 24, 1836. https://encyclopediavirginia.org/entries/horrible-tragedy-raleigh-register-and-north-carolina-gazette-may-24-1836/

5. Messner SF, Baller RD, Zevenbergen MP. The legacy of lynching and southern homicide. *Am Sociol Rev.* 2005;70(4):633–655. https://www.jstor.org/stable/4145380?seq=1

6. Ryan G, Tolnay S. The legacy of lynching? An empirical replication and conceptual extension. *Sociol Spectrum.* 2017;37(2):77–96. https://www.tandfonline.com/doi/full/10.1080/02732173.2017.1287614

7. Ward G. Microclimates of racial meaning: Historical racial violence and environmental impacts. *Wisc Law Rev.* 2016;(3):575–626. https://repository.law.wisc.edu/s/uwlaw/item/77173

8. Ward G. Living histories of White supremacist policing: Towards transformative justice. *Du Bois Rev.* 2018;15(1):167–184. https://www.cambridge.org/core/services/aop-cambridge-core/content/view/E2503031AD0D2A85B464E56D44930166/S1742058X18000139a.pdf/div-class-title-living-histories-of-white-supremacist-policing-div.pdf

9. Ward G, Petersen N, Kupchik A, Pratt J. Historic lynching and corporal punishment in contemporary southern schools. *Soc Probl.* 2021;68(1):41–62. https://academic.oup.com/socpro/article-abstract/68/1/41/5628172?redirectedFrom=fulltext

10. Ward G. *Truths and Reckonings: The Art of Transformative Racial Justice.* St. Louis, Mo.: Mildred Lane Kemper Art Museum, 2020. https://issuu.com/gward-wustl/docs/ward_tg_catalogue_compressedprint

11. Child Opportunity Index. Diversity Data Kids, 2021. https://www.diversitydatakids.org/child-opportunity-index

12. Reece J, Martin M, Bates J, et al. History matters: Understanding the role of policy, race and real estate in today's geography of health equity and opportunity in Cuyahoga County. Cuyahoga County PlaceMatters. February 2015. https://kirwaninstitute.osu.edu/research/cuyahoga-placematters-history-matters-report

13. Reece J. Confronting the legacy of "separate but equal": Can the history of race, real estate, and discrimination engage and inform contemporary policy? *Russell Sage Foundation Journal of the Social Sciences.* 2021;7(1):110–133. https://www.rsfjournal.org/content/7/1/110

14. Reece et al., 2015.

15. Reece et al., 2015.

16. *Clarion Ledger,* Jackson, Miss., 2001.

17. Pettus EW. Mississippi man takes Confederate flag fight to high court." *AP News.* June 28, 2017. https://apnews.com/article/73b8172f60db4fe9b42990074665a91f

18. Orey BD, Baptist N, Sinclair-Chapman V. Racial identity and emotional responses to Confederate symbols. *Social Science Quarterly.* 2021;102(4):1882–1893. https://onlinelibrary.wiley.com/doi/abs/10.1111/ssqu.13032

19. Bieler D. Star Mississippi State RB threatens to leave program unless state changes its flag. *Washington Post.* June 23, 2020. https://www.washingtonpost.com/sports/2020/06/23/star-mississippi-state-rb-threatens-leave-program-unless-state-changes-its-flag/

20. *From Heritage to Health: A Health Impact Assessment Approach to the Adams County Civil Rights Project.* Jackson, Miss.: Mississippi State Department of Health, 2019. http://www.msdh.state.ms.us/msdhsite/index.cfm/44,8319,236,63,pdf/AdamsCounty HealthAssessment.pdf

21. *From Heritage to Health,* 2019, pp. 70–71.

22. Wells J. A "monumental announcement"—it's time we honor our US Colored Troops. ListenUpYall.com. April 8, 2021. https://listenupyall.com/2021/04/08/a-monumental-announcement-its-time-we-honor-our-us-colored-troops/

23. The 1619 Project Curriculum. Washington, D.C.: The Pulitzer Center. https://pulitzercenter.org/lesson-plan-grouping/1619-project-curriculum

24. Rodriguez B. Republican state lawmakers want to punish schools that teach the 1619 Project. *USA Today.* February 10, 2021. https://www.usatoday.com/story/news/education/2021/02/10/slavery-and-history-states-threaten-funding-schools-teach-1619-project/4454195001/

25. The 1619 Project. *New York Times Magazine*. August 14, 2019. https://www.nytimes.com/interactive/2019/08/14/magazine/1619-america-slavery.html

Spotlight

1. Gregg EW, Zhuo X, Cheng Y, et al. Trends in lifetime risk and years of life lost due to diabetes in the USA, 1985–2011: A modelling study. *Lancet Diabetes Endocrinol*. 2014;2(11):8670874. *https://www.sciencedirect.com/science/article/abs/pii/S2213858714701615*

2. Harris JL, Frazier III W, Kumanyika S, Ramirez AG. *Increasing Disparities in Unhealthy Food Advertising Targeted to Hispanic and Black Youth*. UConn Rudd Center for Food Policy & Obesity, 2019.

Chapter 9

1. The term "opportunity hoarding" was coined by Charles Tilly in 1998. See: Tilly C. How to hoard opportunities. *Durable Inequality*. Berkeley and Los Angeles: University of California Press, 1998:147–169. *https://gsdrc.org/document-library/how-to-hoard-opportunities/*

2. RWJF grant ID 71192, Establishing an Information System to Track and Study Child Health, Well-Being, and Equity, October 1, 2013, to September 30, 2017, $2,895,539. *https://www.rwjf.org/en/how-we-work/grants-explorer.html#k=diversitydatakids.org*

3. RWJF grant ID 75969, Enhancing the Ability to Understand and Spread the Child Opportunity Index's Impact in Creating Equitable Access to Healthy Communities for Kids, December 1, 2018, to November 30, 2021, $2,996,123. *https://www.rwjf.org/en/how-we-work/grants-explorer.html#k=child%20opportunity%20index*

4. Noelke C, McArdle N, Baek M, et al. Child Opportunity Index 2.0: Technical Documentation. diversitydatakids.org, 2020. *https://www.diversitydatakids.org/sites/default/files/2020-02/ddk_coi2.0_technical_documentation_20200212.pdf*

5. Child Opportunity Index (COI). diversitydatakids.org, 2020. *https://www.diversitydatakids.org/child-opportunity-index*

6. Lo L. Who zones? Mapping land-use authority across the US. Urban Wire: Neighborhoods, Cities, and Metros, Urban Institute blog. December 9, 2019. *https://www.urban.org/urban-wire/who-zones-mapping-land-use-authority-across-us*

7. Hoyt H, Schuetz J. *Parking requirements and foundations are driving up the cost of multifamily housing*. Brookings Institution. 2020. *https://www.brookings.edu/research/parking-requirements-and-foundations-are-driving-up-the-cost-of-multifamily-housing/*

8. *Mount Laurel Doctrine*. Fair Share Housing Center. *https://fairsharehousing.org/mount-laurel-doctrine/*

9. The Mount Laurel Doctrine. *New York Times*. January 28, 2013. *https://www.nytimes.com/2013/01/29/opinion/the-mount-laurel-doctrine.html*

10. Massey DS, Albright L, Casciano R, et al. *Climbing Mount Laurel: The Struggle for Affordable Housing and Social Mobility in an American Suburb*. Princeton, NJ: Princeton University Press, 2013. *https://press.princeton.edu/books/hardcover/9780691157290/climbing-mount-laurel*

11. Chetty R, Hendren N, Katz L. The effects of exposure to better neighborhoods on children: New evidence from the Moving to Opportunity Experiment. *Am Econ Rev*. 2016;106(4):855–902. *https://opportunityinsights.org/paper/newmto/*

12. Low-income housing tax credits. National Housing Law Project. 2017. *https://www.nhlp.org/resource-center/low-income-housing-tax-credits/*

13. Source of income laws by state, county and city. National Multifamily Housing Council. February 1, 2021. *https://www.nmhc.org/research-insight/analysis-and-guidance/source-of-income-laws-by-state-county-and-city/*

14. Memorandum on redressing our nation's and the federal government's history of discriminatory housing practices and policies. Memorandum for the Secretary of Housing and Urban Development, The White House. January 26, 2021. *https://www.whitehouse.gov/briefing-room/presidential-actions/2021/01/26/memorandum-on-redressing-our-nations-and-the-federal-governments-history-of-discriminatory-housing-practices-and-policies/*

15. President Biden signs American Rescue Plan Act with nearly $50 billion in housing and homelessness assistance. National Low Income Housing Coalition: Memo to Members. March 15, 2021. *https://nlihc.org/resource/ president-biden-signs-american-rescue-plan-act-nearly-50-billion-housing-and-homelessness*

Chapter 10

1. Van Helden A, Harden D. You Don't Know Me. Song on studio album *2 Future 4 U*, released January 25, 1999. Music track by Armand Van Helden, lyrics and vocals by Duane Harden. *https://www.youtube.com/watch?v=yNSpLqmY6K0*
2. Alkin MC, King JA. The historical development of evaluation use. *Am J Eval.* 2016;37(4):568– 579. *https://escholarship.org/content/qt2qn5x84t/qt2qn5x84t_noSplash_4e4529f18e9a5777 3f3766c546aa4d2d.pdf*
3. Weiss CH. Utilization of evaluation: Toward comparative study. In Weiss CH (Ed.), *Evaluating Action Programs: Readings in Social Action and Education.* Boston: Allyn and Bacon, 1972:318–326.
4. Dean-Coffey J. What's race got to do with it? Equity and philanthropic evaluation practice. *Am J Eval.* 2018;39(4):527–542. *https://journals.sagepub.com/doi/pdf/10.1177/ 1098214018778533*
5. About Equitable Evaluation Initiative. Equitable Evaluation Initiative, 2021. *https://www. equitableeval.org/about*
6. For more on the history of philanthropy arising from a White-dominant culture intent on protecting its wealth, see: Villanueva E. *Decolonizing Wealth: Indigenous Wisdom to Health Divides and Restore Balance.* Penguin Random House, 2018. New York, New York *https:// www.penguinrandomhouse.com/books/588996/decolonizing-wealth-by-edgar-villanueva/*.
7. For more on addressing the effects of the White-dominant philanthropic history and culture, see: Johnson M, Chen A. A call-in to grow indigenous power. *Stanford Social Innovation Review.* March 11, 2021. *https://ssir.org/articles/entry/a_call_in_to_grow_indigenous_power#*
8. About Equitable Evaluation Initiative.
9. Equitable Evaluation Framework™. Equitable Evaluation Initiative, 2021. *https://www. equitableeval.org/framework*
10. Center for Evaluation Innovation, Institute for Foundation and Donor Learning, Dorothy A. Johnson Center for Philanthropy, Luminare Group. Equitable Evaluation Framing Paper. Equitable Evaluation Initiative, July 2017. *www.equitableeval.org*
11. Equitable Evaluation Framework™.
12. Ortiz Aragón A, Hoetmer R. Flowing with the river's go: Seeking ethical, pragmatic, and strategic participation in the design of a regional funding strategy. *Int Rev Qual Res.* 2020;13(2):112–139. *https://journals.sagepub.com/doi/abs/10.1177/1940844720933217*
13. Stringer ET, Ortiz Aragón A. *Action Research*, 5th ed. Thousand Oaks, CA: Sage Publishing, 2021. *https://us.sagepub.com/en-us/nam/action-research/book266023*
14. Addressing Community Health and Well-Being Issues in San Antonio, Texas, Through Culturally Responsive and Participatory Approaches. RWJF Grant ID 77372, April 15, 2020, to September 14, 2021. *https://www.rwjf.org/en/how-we-work/grants-explorer.html#k= University%20of%20the%20Incarnate%20Word*
15. Stringer ET, Ortiz Aragón A. *Action Research*, 5th ed. Thousand Oaks, CA: Sage Publishing, 2021. *https://us.sagepub.com/en-us/nam/action-research/book266023*
16. Reeler D. A Theory of Social Change and Implications for Practice, Planning, Monitoring and Evaluation. Community Development Resource Association, 2007. *http://www. managingforimpact.org/sites/default/files/resource/a_theory_of_social_change_and_ implications.pdf*
17. Mertens DM. *Research and Evaluation in Education and Psychology: Integrating Diversity with Quantitative, Qualitative, and Mixed Methods*, 5th ed. Thousand Oaks, CA: Sage, 2020; Mertens DM, Wilson AT. *Program Evaluation Theory and Practice: A Comprehensive Approach*, 2nd ed. New York: Guilford, 2019; Mertens DM. *Mixed Methods Design in Evaluation.* Thousand Oaks, CA: Sage, 2018.

18. Bolinson C, Mertens D. A Transformative Evaluation Toolkit for the Impact Investing Sector. Engineers Without Borders Canada, September 2019. Toronto, Canada *https://www.ewb.ca/wp-content/uploads/2019/10/Tool-Kit-document-Interactive_FINAL_Oct31.pdf*

19. Bolinson C, Mertens DM. Transformative evaluation and impact investing: A fruitful marriage. In Herman RP, de Morais Sarmento E (Eds.), *Global Handbook of Impact Investing*. Wiley, 2020.

20. Chilisa B, Mertens DM. Indigenous made in Africa evaluation frameworks: Addressing epistemic violence and contributing to social transformation. *Am J Eval.* 2021;42(2):241–253. *https://journals.sagepub.com/doi/full/10.1177/1098214020948601*

Spotlight

1. Using Health Data for New York City in Advancing Policy-Relevant Research to Promote Health Equity. RWJF Grant ID 75962; $993,425; November 15, 2018, to May 15, 2021. *https://www.rwjf.org/en/how-we-work/grants-explorer.html#k=New%20York%20City%20Department%20of%20Health%20and%20Mental%20Hygiene*

Chapter 11

1. NAACP. About us. *https://naacp.org/about-us/* Accessed January 25, 2021.

2. National Archives. Black Americans and the vote. *https://www.archives.gov/research/african-americans/vote*

3. USA.gov. Voting and election laws. *https://www.usa.gov/voting-laws*

4. OurDocuments.gov. 19th Amendment to the U.S. Constitution: Women's Right to Vote (1920). *https://www.ourdocuments.gov/doc.php?flash=false&doc=63*

5. 2020 Women's Vote Centennial Initiative. FAQs. *https://www.2020centennial.org/faq*

6. Library of Congress. Voting rights for Native Americans. *https://www.loc.gov/classroom-materials/elections/right-to-vote/voting-rights-for-native-americans/*

7. NPR. Yes, women could vote after the 19th Amendment—but not all women. Or men. *https://www.npr.org/2020/08/26/904730251/yes-women-could-vote-after-the-19th-amendment-but-not-all-women-or-men*

8. Uggen C, Larson R, Shannon S, Pulido-Nava A. Locked Out 2020: Estimates of people denied voting rights due to a felony conviction. The Sentencing Project. October 30, 2020. *https://www.sentencingproject.org/publications/locked-out-2020-estimates-of-people-denied-voting-rights-due-to-a-felony-conviction/*

9. National Conference of State Legislatures. Felon voting rights. *https://www.ncsl.org/research/elections-and-campaigns/felon-voting-rights.aspx* Accessed January 27, 2021.

10. National Conference of State Legislatures, 2021.

11. National Archives. Congress and the Voting Rights Act of 1965. *https://www.archives.gov/legislative/features/voting-rights-1965*

12. Brennan Center for Justice. The effects of *Shelby County v. Holder.* August 6, 2018. *https://www.brennancenter.org/our-work/policy-solutions/effects-shelby-county-v-holder*

13. *https://www.usatoday.com/in-depth/news/politics/elections/2021/01/06/trumps-failed-efforts-overturn-election-numbers/4130307001/*

14. Krebs C. Opinion: Trump fired me for saying this, but I'll say it again: The election wasn't rigged. *Washington Post.* December 1, 2020. *https://www.washingtonpost.com/opinions/christopher-krebs-trump-election-wasnt-hacked/2020/12/01/88da94a0-340f-11eb-8d38-6aea1adb3839_story.html*

15. Brennan Center for Justice. *Brnovich v. Democratic National Committee.* January 19, 2021. *https://www.brennancenter.org/our-work/court-cases/brnovich-v-democratic-national-committee*

16. Ura A. Gov. Greg Abbott signs Texas voting bill into law, overcoming Democratic quorum breaks. September 7, 2021. *https://www.texastribune.org/2021/09/01/texas-voting-bill-greg-abbott/*

17. NPR. Robocalls, rumors and emails: Last-minute election disinformation floods voters. October 24, 2020. *https://www.npr.org/2020/10/24/927300432/robocalls-rumors-and-emails-last-minute-election-disinformation-floods-voters*

18. Massingale BN. The racist attack on our nation's Capitol. *America: The Jesuit Review.* January 6, 2021. *https://www.americamagazine.org/politics-society/2021/01/06/us-capitol-trump-riot-racist-239662*

19. Brennan Center for Justice. Voting laws roundup: July 2021. July 22, 2021. *https://www.brennancenter.org/our-work/research-reports/voting-laws-roundup-july-2021*

20. Census Counts 2020. *https://censuscounts.org*

21. Constitution Annotated. ArtI.S2.C3.1 Enumeration Clause. *https://constitution.congress.gov/browse/essay/artI-S2-C3-1/ALDE_00001034/*

22. *https://www.census.gov/programs-surveys/decennial-census/decade/2020/about.html.* Accessed March 3, 2022.

23. National Archives and Records Administration. African Americans and the Federal Census, 1790–1930. *https://www.archives.gov/files/research/census/african-american/census-1790-1930.pdf*

24. U.S. Census Bureau. Censuses of American Indians. *https://www.census.gov/history/www/genealogy/decennial_census_records/censuses_of_american_indians.html* Accessed January 29, 2021.

25. U.S. Census Bureau. 2020 Census. *https://2020census.gov/content/dam/2020census/materials/partners/2020-06/CENSUS-COUNTS-EVERYONE_en.pdfad*

26. U.S. Census Bureau. What we do. *https://www.census.gov/about/what.html* Accessed January 29, 2021.

27. GW Institute of Public Policy, George Washington University. Counting for dollars 2020: The role of the decennial census in the geographic distribution of federal funds. *https://gwipp.gwu.edu/counting-dollars-2020-role-decennial-census-geographic-distribution-federal-funds#Resources%20for%20Journalists*

28. Macagnone M. Polls: Most people still think census will ask about citizenship. Roll Call. February 20, 2020. *https://www.rollcall.com/2020/02/20/polls-most-people-still-think-census-will-ask-about-citizenship/*

29. NPR. How Trump officials cut the 2020 Census short amid the pandemic. September 18, 2020. *https://www.npr.org/2020/09/18/911960963/how-trump-officials-cut-the-2020-census-short-amid-the-pandemic*

30. Schneider M. Supreme Court halts census in latest twist of 2020 count. Associated Press. October 14, 2020. *https://apnews.com/article/us-news-census-2020-c6cb554611d328b423ac508e5008f9cd*

31. Epstein B, Lofquist D. U.S. Census Bureau today delivers state population totals for Congressional apportionment. U.S. Census Bureau. April 26, 2021. *https://www.census.gov/library/stories/2021/04/2020-census-data-release.html*

32. National Conference of State Legislatures. 2020 Census delays and the impact on redistricting. September 23, 2021. *https://www.ncsl.org/research/redistricting/2020-census-delays-and-the-impact-on-redistricting-637261879.aspx*

33. U.S. Census Bureau. Race. *https://www.census.gov/quickfacts/fact/note/US/RHI625219#:~:text=Asian.-,A%20person%20having%20origins%20in%20any%20of%20the%20original%20peoples,Islands%2C%20Thailand%2C%20and%20Vietnam* Accessed January 29, 2021.

34. U.S. Census Bureau. Race.

35. The word "Asians" is used in accordance with the presentation in the American Community Survey.

36. U.S. Census Bureau. About the American Community Survey. *https://www.census.gov/programs-surveys/acs/about.html*

37. U.S. Census Bureau. American Community Survey Demographic and Housing Estimates, Table DP05 (ACS 2017 1-Year estimate vs 2010 1-Year estimate). *https://data.census.gov/cedsci/table?q=2019%20ACS%201-Year&tid=ACSDP1Y2019.DP05&hidePreview=true*

38. *Ibid.*

39. U.S. Census Bureau. 2020 Census Barriers, Attitudes, and Motivators Study Survey Report: A New Design for the 21st Century. January 24, 2019. *https://www2.census.gov/programs-surveys/decennial/2020/program-management/final-analysis-reports/2020-report-cbams-study-survey.pdf*

40. The word "Hispanics" is used in accordance with the presentation in the Census Barriers, Attitudes, and Motivators Study.

41. Runes C, Park Y. Census 2020: Ensuring "hard-to-count" Asian Americans count at the federal, state, and local levels. Urban Institute. *https://www.urban.org/urban-wire/census-2020-ensuring-hard-count-asian-americans-count-federal-state-and-local-levels* Accessed January 30, 2021.

42. Ruiz NG, Menasce Horowitz J, Tamir C. Many Black and Asian Americans say they have experienced discrimination amid the COVID-19 outbreak. Pew Research Center. July 1, 2020. *https://www.pewsocialtrends.org/2020/07/01/many-black-and-asian-americans-say-they-have-experienced-discrimination-amid-the-covid-19-outbreak*

43. Yi SS, Kwon SC, Sacks R, Trinh-Shevrin C. Commentary: Persistence and health-related consequences of the model minority stereotype for Asian Americans. *Ethn Dis.* 2016;26(1):133–138. *https://www.ncbi.nlm.nih.gov/pmc/articles/PMC4738850/*

44. NPR. For the U.S. Census, keeping your data anonymous and useful is a tricky balance. August 2, 2021. *https://www.npr.org/2021/05/19/993247101/for-the-u-s-census-keeping-your-data-anonymous-and-useful-is-a-tricky-balance*

45. *https://www.raceforward.org/press/releases/national-racial-justice-organizations-join-together-map-hardest-count-communities*

Epilogue

1. Carman KG, Chandra A, Bugliari D, et al. COVID-19 and the Experiences of Populations at Greater Risk. RAND Corporation, Social and Economic Well-Being Division, sponsored by the Robert Wood Johnson Foundation. Fall 2020.

2. *Building Community Power to Advance Health Equity,* a RWJF Collection.

3. RWJF commits $50 million for immediate COVID-19 relief. *Philanthropy News Digest.* April 9, 2020.

4. Besser R. Letter to the Members of the Board of Trustees, the Robert Wood Johnson Foundation, July 17, 2020.

5. Robert Wood Johnson Foundation provides $50 million to support those facing greatest strain under the COVID-19 pandemic. *RWJF.* April 7, 2020.

6. *Building Community Power to Advance Health Equity.*

7. *Building Community Power to Advance Health Equity.*

8. Besser R, Stewart S. To end America's maternal mortality crisis, dismantle the racism that fuels it. *CNN Opinion.* July 14, 2021.

9. RWJF Board Book. *Increasing Community Power.* October 2020.

10. Christopher G, Plough A. New commission to tackle how national health data are collected, shared, and used. Health Affairs. May 18, 2021. https://www.healthaffairs.org/do/10.1377/forefront.20210518.409206/full/

11. Christopher GC, Zimmerman EB, Chandra A., Martin LT. Charting a course for an equity-centered data system: Recommendations from the National Commission to Transform Public Health Data Systems. RWJF. October 19, 2021. *https://www.rwjf.org/en/library/research/2021/10/charting-a-course-for-an-equity-centered-data-system.html*

12. Executive Summary and Introduction, first report of the National Commission to Transform Public Health Data, Fall 2021.

13. RWJF Grant ID No. 76915, Advancing culture change for increased social justice, health, and equity by working through the popular entertainment media.

14. RWJF Grant ID No. 76323, USC Center for Health Journalism, National Fellowship.

15. Health & Hollywood: Putting a little spinach in the popcorn. *RWJF Culture of Health Blog.* October 31, 2011 https://www.rwjf.org/en/blog/2011/10/health-hollywood-putting-a-little-spinach-in-the-popcorn.html. Also RWJF Grant ID. No. 76763, Examining the feasibility of investing in the creative community to imagine popular storylines to inspire a Culture of Health mindset in America.

16. Stripling J. How Chapel Hill bungled a star hire. Chronicle of Higher Education. July 6, 2021. *https://www.chronicle.com/article/how-chapel-hill-bungled-a-star-hire*

Spotlight

1. Vaidya A. Walk with us: Building community power and connection for health equity. RWJF Culture of Health Blog. August 20, 2019. https://www.rwjf.org/en/blog/2019/08/walk-with-us--building-community-power-and-connection-for-health-equity.html
2. Vaidya, 2019.
3. Braverman P, Arkin E, Orleans T, et al. What is health equity? RWJF. May 1, 2017. *https://www.rwjf.org/en/library/research/2017/05/what-is-health-equity-.html*

INDEX